MODERN
Instrumental
Delivery

MODERN
Instrumental
Delivery

JOHN PATRICK O'GRADY, M.D.

Chief, Division of Maternal-Fetal Medicine
MacDonald Hospital for Women
Associate Professor
Department of Reproduction Biology
Case Western Reserve University
Cleveland, Ohio

Illustrations prepared by
NANCY A. BURGARD, M.A.

WILLIAMS & WILKINS
Baltimore • Hong Kong • London • Sydney

Editor: Carol-Lynn Brown
Associate Editor: Victoria M. Vaughn
Copy Editor: Klemie Bryte
Design: Norman W. Och
Illustration Planning: Wayne Hubbel
Production: Theda Harris
Cover Design: Bob Och

Copyright ©1988
Williams & Wilkins
428 East Preston Street
Baltimore, MD 21202, U.S.A.

Printed in the United States of America

Main entry under title:

Library of Congress Cataloging-in-Publication Data
O'Grady, John Patrick, 1945-
  Modern instrumental delivery.

  Includes index.
  1. Forceps, obstetric.   2. Obstetrical extraction.
I. Title.   [DNLM: 1. Delivery—methods.   2. Extraction,
obstetrical.   3. Obstetrical forceps. WQ 415 035m]
RG739.037   1988   618.8'2'028   87-29562
ISBN 0-683-06632-3

88 89 90 91 92 10 9 8 7 6 5 4 3 2 1

To J.O., who always
wanted his son to be a surgeon
and to J.A. Morris, M.D.,
who taught me how.

Plus ça change, plus c'est la même chose.
Alphonse Karr
Les Guêpes, 1849

PREFACE

The use of instruments to assist delivery has a long and often colorful history. Obstetric forceps designed to assist delivery of an undamaged child were an invention of the 17th century; however, forceps were maintained as a trade secret by the Chamberlen family for more than 75 years and were not in general use until after 1720. Prior to the development of obstetric forceps various devices were described to assist delivery in complicated cases. Sadly, most, if not all, of these instruments were designed for fetal dismemberment or cranial destruction, as at the time cesarean delivery implied unacceptable maternal morbidity and mortality.

Assisted delivery in obstetrics has always been controversial. From the inception of use of forceps various practitioners argued against their use, citing grave maternal and fetal injuries that might befall when such instruments were applied. Little has changed, at least in this regard. Forceps are still in use, although indications have changed along with obstetric practice. The few difficult or heroic forceps procedures have progressively disappeared, which is all to the good. In recent years, the preponderance of learned opinion has proposed abandonment of forceps procedures—especially midforceps applications—with greater reliance on the stimulation of labor, attentive observation, and cesarean delivery. Cesarean delivery has shown a remarkable increase since 1970 and presently accounts for nearly 20% of deliveries in the United States. In this era of conservatism in use of instrumental vaginal delivery, many practitioners and students are uncertain which procedures are appropriate, safe, and, inevitably, medicolegally defensible. Thus, new, comprehensive review of instrumental delivery is in order. The current text is designed as both a reference and clinical guide. Due to changes in American practice, a review of the vacuum extractor is included. In my opinion, modern accoucheurs should thoroughly understand the use of both types of instruments.

Instrumental delivery requires the greatest diligence and skill on the part of the practitioner. While accoucheurs of only moderate ability can adequately perform cesarean delivery, the requirements for judicious application of force, knowledge of the physiology of labor, and understanding of pelvic anatomy make forceps delivery and, to a lesser extent, vacuum extraction substantially more taxing procedures.

As always, knowing when to intervene is equally as critical as possessing the skill to intervene.

Instrumental delivery is not learned from textbooks, regardless of how gifted or persuasive the author. Instrumental deliveries are a skill—part of the art of obstetrics—that can be studied or discussed but must be experienced at the delivery table with the assistance of a good teacher. Both the forceps and the ventouse are imperfect instruments and can injure mother and child if not used with care. The aim herein is to assist practitioners and students to better understand these instruments and improve their skills.

ACKNOWLEDGMENTS

The preparation of this book was assisted by many. The critique and review of chapters by my colleagues at MacDonald Hospital for Women is gratefully appreciated. My research assistants, John Gazzara, Dan Haghighi, and Kris Napier, Ph.D., contributed long hours and ran down many obscure and unusual requests. Their efforts are recalled with appreciation. The assistance of the Allen Memorial Medical Library staff is gratefully acknowledged. The personnel from the Howard Dittrick Museum of Historical Medicine, especially Glen Jenkins, Judy Chelnick, and James Edmonson, Ph.D., gave generously of their time and expertise. Their contributions to this endeavor were substantial. Finally, special recognition is due to Michelle Maurer for her exceptional loyalty and encouragement throughout this project and for expert assistance in the preparation of the numerous drafts and revisions of this manuscript.

CONTENTS

INTRODUCTION
AND *COUP D'OEIL*: INSTRUMENTAL DELIVERY

The basics of parturition remain unchanged despite technical advances in obstetric practice. Spontaneous and voluntary powers move a passenger through a series of bony and muscular passages to delivery. We can prod or biopsy the fetal passenger, and we know a good deal about the dynamics of *in utero* growth and development. Yet, the subtle interaction between the fetus and birth canal during delivery represents a complex, dynamic mechanism that is still not entirely understood. As a cynic might observe, the phenomenon has remained the same but our explanations for it have changed. Today we can better evaluate the status of the fetus through this journey than our predecessors, but we are not necessarily better clinicians.

The unaided human birth process is not perfect. Further, obstetric interventions including cesarean section are not invariably benign procedures for the mother and do not guarantee a normal child. There will always be a need for instrumental delivery either for fetal distress or to assist in cases of inertia or maternal exhaustion. Even if forceps or vacuum extractor applications were restricted only to instances of fetal distress and outlet procedures, the same considerations of application and technique as needed for more taxing procedures would apply. What is required is a balanced view of risks and benefits when any means of assisted delivery is chosen. The response to either dystocia or apparent fetal distress is not necessarily either cesarean section or instrumental delivery and nonoperative options including observation, stimulation of labor, encouragement, and maternal repositioning must always be considered.

Those speaking as the pacesetters for obstetric practice throughout the turbulent history of instrumental delivery have always had mixed feelings about the use of forceps or the vacuum extractor. In the first few decades following the discovery of forceps, little criticism was voiced. The need for a method of assisted delivery was so acute that the inevitable complications of instrumentation were viewed as a lesser evil than either fetal destruction or maternal death. However, in the early decades of the 19th century, conservatism and "leaving to nature" returned in obstetric practice, partially in response to the excesses of forceps use with their inevitable toll of damaged mothers and damaged or destroyed infants (1). The popularity of instrumental delivery has also reflected trends in society as well. Instrumentation became popular again in the latter half of the 19th century. Rapid changes in obstetric practice were instituted in a period when the prevalent view in society was that invention meant improvement and that technology was the path to the future. In the early decades of the 20th century, the concept of "prophylactic forceps" fit in well with the idea of delivery as a surgical, scientific procedure best conducted in a hospital setting. Routine instrumentation was finally run aground in recent years when a new backlash against instrumental assistance developed. What is unclear is whether the pendulum will swing back and whether instrumental delivery will again become popular. A selection of quotations follows, illustrating the controversial and colorful history of medical instrumentation.

It is unfortunate that there is no law to punish ignorant physicians, and that capital punishment is never inflicted upon them. Yet they learn by our suffering and they experiment by putting us to death. (Pliny, The Elder, 79 AD) (2)

If the fetus does not respond to manual traction, because of its size, or death, or impaction in any manner whatsoever, one must proceed to the more forceful methods, those of extraction by hooks and embryotomy. For even if one loses the infant, it is still necessary to take care of the mother. (Soranus, ca. 100 AD) (3)

. . . then it came to the day of their birth, and the maiden named Bloodwoman gave birth . . . they were born suddenly. Two of them were born, named Hunahpu and Xbalanque. . . . (Popol Vuh ca. 300–500 AD) (4)

The more types of these instruments the practitioner has ready by him, the more rapidly he operates, and the greater his reputation among men. So do not neglect to have ready by you a single one of these instruments, for you will certainly need it. (Albucasis, 1010 AD) (5)

. . . I have been wont for so many years, frequently and with God Almighty's assistance, to help women in difficult labors, . . . Indeed, the most important point lies in the conformation of the pubic bones themselves as they are first formed . . . the parts of the parturient become so narrow that the road is not wide enough for the fetus, . . . But when matters have become so difficult and have reached the point that grave danger threatens and that we remain in doubt about the child, whether it might live or die— what then should a Christian physician do and what resolution should he form? For if he leaves the patient without help, he will acquire the reputation of being inhuman. If on the other hand he rationally employs . . . dismembering instruments and kills the fetus which perchance is still alive, and has not been ablouted from the sacred font, so that the woman may be saved, he will burden his own conscience since evil should never be done that good may result. And he will have to render an account of his stewardship to the Highest . . . since it usually happens that, due to the very difficulty of the work and its long duration, the strength of the mother gives out during the operation and malicious accusation of the art arises. (Gulio Caesare Aranzi (Aratius), 1564) (6)

My Father, Brothers and Myself . . . have by God's Blessing and our Industry . . . practiced a way to deliver Women in this case without any prejudice to them or their Infants. (Hugh Chamberlen, Sr., 1696) (7)

As to the forceps, which, I think no person has yet anymore than barely mentioned, it is a noble instrument, to which many now living owe their lives, as I can assert from my own knowledge and long successful practice. (Edmund Chapman, 1735) (8)

The use of instruments is sometimes needful, not withstanding any arguments to the contrary, but the too free use of them ought by no means to be encouraged. They are sometimes unnecessarily applied, and are frequently productive of great mischief; but many lives, not only of mothers, but of children have been saved by them, of which every one must be sensible, who has been much versed in general practice. (Charles White, 1777) (9)

By not meeting with the attention which it merits . . . forceps . . . are daily employed with too much freedom, to the disgrace of the Art and often with irreparable injury to mother and child. (Benjamin Bell, 1789) (10)

The general arguments against the use of instruments have been drawn from their abuse; it appears, however, that necessity will justify the use of the forceps; that when such necessity exists, their use is not only justifiable, but often highly advantageous; (however,) that delay to apply them, and slowness in their application and use, will secure, as far as possible, both the mother and child from untoward accidents; but that mischief cannot be prevented if they are applied too soon, or the operations with them be performed in a hurry. (T. Denman, 1803) (11)

Obstetric operations should perhaps never be undertaken excepting as a means of diminishing or of removing some well-marked or strongly apprehended cause of danger, either to the mother or her progeny. Hence it follows, that, whenever an obstetric operation of any consequence is JUDICIOUSLY proposed, it is to be assumed that there is danger, either present or apprehended, to be obviated by it. But to this assumption of existing danger, must also be added a certain contingent risk of danger to be incurred by the operation itself: and it were, indeed, well for the credit of the art, if this latter source of danger should be estimated as of trifling importance in comparison of it with the former. (D.D. Davis, 1834) (12)

The question then arises, "Should instruments ever be used?" To which I reply—I would not say that there was no case in which they were admissible; but this I would state, that the cases in which it is ever justifiable to use them are exceedingly rare; and that instrumental delivery should never be attempted until all the means recommended to alleviate the sufferings and expedite the birth under difficult, preternatural, and complex labors, have been tried in vain. And if so, I believe that, with most practitioners, instruments will become as rusty as did those of Dr. Hunter, of London. (W. Beach, 1847) (13)

... In giving this advice, we doubtless will fall under the censure of those who pour their anathemas upon what they call "meddlesome midwifery" which expression, although it may serve as a caveat to the ignorant and rash, the author has always regarded as an evidence that those who employ it are themselves ignorant alike of the extent of the resources of nature and those also in science; and, hence, "trusting to nature" until the danger to the child and parent are so cumulative that artificial assistance; tardily rendered is not only unavailing, but often accessory to a fatal determination. He who understands accurately the natural modes of delivery, and the resources of his science, may enjoy the unspeakable pleasure of diminishing corporal and mental suffering in a very large number of these cases ... and very often of preserving lives which would otherwise have been sacrificed. (H.L. Hodge, 1864) (14)

But again we are told that the forceps is a dangerous instrument. ... The effect of all this has been in the minds of many to make the use of the forceps an act which carries with it a large degree of impropriety, and even may make one ashamed of his doing. When, therefore, under the inspiration of such mental hesitancy, one takes up the dreaded instrument, doubt seizes on him, and may unman him and unfit him for the emergency he is facing; he is confirmed in his preconceived (because so taught) ideas, and he abandons the attempt in confusion, or blindly gropes his way through with a lively but not very comforting apprehension of the horrors in store for the unfortunate patient. ... It is the abuse and not the use of the instrument that does harm, and the best way to obviate this evil is to train our young men to greater skill, show them how to rightly use the instrument, and give them the confidence in the work they are undertaking. (E.S. Dunster, 1877) (15)

... d'ouvrir un aneurysme, pour un abcès, ne pouvre rien contre bistouri! (C. Pajot, 1882) (16)

"The prophylactic forceps operation" is the routine delivery of the child in head presentation when the head has come to rest on the pelvic floor, ... it is not a complete reversal of the watchful expectancy that is universally taught, but I cannot deny that it interferes much with Nature's process. Were not the results I have achieved so gratifying, I myself would call it meddlesome midwifery. For unskilled hands it is unjustifiable ... One may well ask himself whether the brief and moderate compression of the head and the skillfully performed forceps operation, is not less dangerous to the integrity of the brain than the prolonged pounding and congestion it suffers from a hard spontaneous delivery. If a late forceps operation is done on a head and a brain already infiltrated with small hemorrhages, the results are worse, compounded. (J.B. DeLee, 1920) (17)

From the obstetrical forceps, good Lord, deliver us! (Sir C. Berkeley, 1923) (18)

The amount of traction which can be exerted by the forceps, especially axis traction forceps, is enormous, because, if well applied, the blades grasp the head so exactly. It is perfection of design which makes the obstetric forceps such a dangerous instrument in the hands of the inexperienced and aggressive accoucheur, who does not appreciate his own limitations and the limitations of the instrument. I have seen an accoucheur with his feet up against the couch, even applied to the buttocks of the patient, exerting all his strength. I have occasionally exerted a considerable amount of force myself, although I believe this is seldom justified. The instrument is, then, as a rule, being used in a wrong manner, or too early, or is unsuitable in the particular circumstances. (J.M.M. Kerr, 1937) (19)

It must be recognized, however, that just as long as a forceps operation is dependent upon individual judgement, disasters are inevitable and the obstetrical forceps will continue to take their toll of life and well being. The instrument is not infrequently used under conditions which require the application of what most authorities describe as "tentative traction,"... Unfortunately, the estimation of tentative traction depends entirely on individual judgement—a purely human faculty subject to the variation and error of all human attributes... if delivery is possible with brute strength, it can always be more safely accomplished by knowledge and art. (J. Baxter, 1946) (20)

Strictly speaking, the termination of labor by forceps, provided it can be accomplished without great danger, is indicated in any condition which threatens the life of the mother or child, and which offers a reasonable prospect of being relieved by delivery. (N.J. Eastman, 1950) (21)

As to the type of forceps used,... this is not as important as the man behind them ... (A.H. Bill, 1954) (22)

The literature is already replete with grisly accounts of sloughing scalps, intracranial haemorrhages, cephalhaematomata, depressed fracture of the skull, death and destruction which accord ill with our own experience and with that of colleagues of mine in other centers who have acquired a proper experience of the instrument (ventouse). All this has helped to fan the predjudice of reactionary obstetricians, some of whom argued fiercely with me and with apparent intelligence and then finally confessed they had never even seen the instrument used or had certainly not attempted to use it themselves. Tradition dies hard and midwives of both sexes are often remarkable for their conservatism. (I. Donald, 1979) (23)

... the idea that physical violence ... is a common cause of cerebral birth injury, has now been discounted. Indeed, the evidence is that the competent use of instruments ... prevents injury. Where injury occurs in association with a difficult and complicated delivery in which instruments have been used, such use is likely to have prevented even worse damage. (J.O. Forfar, 1984) (24)

It would be absurd to suggest that brain damage cannot occur during labor or delivery; but there is much evidence to suggest that doctors and others are all too ready to ascribe mental subnormality or cerebral palsy to such damage. (R.S. Illingworth, 1985) (25)

REFERENCES

1. Leavitt JW. "Science" enters the birthing room: obstetrics in America since the eighteenth century. J Am Hist 1983; 70:281–303.
2. Guthrie D. A history of medicine. London: Thomas Nelson & Sons, Ltd, 1945.
3. Temkin O, Eastman NJ, Edelstein L, Guttmacher AF. Soranus' Gynecology. Baltimore: Johns Hopkins University Press, 1956: 189–190.
4. Tedlock D [Translator]. Popol Vuh. New York: Simon & Schuster, Inc, 1985: 119.
5. Spink MS, Lewis GL. Albucasis on surgery and instruments. Berkeley: University of California Press, 1973: 494.
6. Aranzi GC. De humano foeto liber, 1564. In: Eastman NJ, ed. Pelvic measuration: a study in the perpetuation of an error. Obstet Gynecol Surv 1948; 3:301–329.
7. Drinkwater KR. The midwifery forceps: historical sketch. Liverpool Medico-Chirurgical J 1913; 64:451–465.
8. Chapman E. A treatise on the improvement of midwifery. London, 1735.
9. White C. Treatise on the management of pregnant and lying-in women, and the means of curing, but more especially of preventing the principle disorders to which they are liable. London: Dilly, 1777.
10. Bell B. System of surgery. 1789.
11. Denman T. Aphorisms on the application and use of forceps and vectis, on preternatural labours, on labours attended by haemorrhage, and with convulsions. Philadelphia: Johnson, 1803.
12. Davis DD. Principles and practice of obstetric medicine. London: Taylor, 1836.
13. Beach W. An improved system of midwifery, New York: Beach, 1847.
14. Hodge HL. The principles and practice of obstetrics, New York, 1864.
15. Dunster ES. The use of obstetric forceps in abbreviating the second stage of labor. Tr Med Soc Mich (Lansing) 1877; 132–133.
16. Pajot C. Travaux d'obstetrique et de gynecologie, précédés d'elements de pratique obstetricale. Paris: H. Lauwereynes, 1882.
17. DeLee JB. The prophylactic forceps operation. Am J Obstet Gynecol 1920; 1:34–44.
18. Berkeley C. The use and abuse of obstetric forceps. J Obstet Gynaecol Br Emp 1923; 30:413–429.
19. Kerr JMM. Operative obstetrics. London: Bailliere, Tindall, & Cox, 1937: 438.
20. Baxter J. The obstetrical forceps: controlled axis traction. J Obstet Gynaecol Br Emp 1946; 53:42–54.
21. Eastman NJ. Williams obstetrics, 10th ed. New York, Appleton-Century-Crofts, 1950: 1057.
22. Bill AH. Forceps delivery. Am J Obstet Gynecol 1954; 68:245–249.
23. Donald I. Practical obstetric problems. 5th ed. London, Lloyd-Luke, 1979: 677.
24. Forfar JO, Arneil JC, eds. Paediatrics. Edinburgh: Churchill Livingstone Co., 1984.
25. Illingworth, RS. A paediatrician asks—why is it called birth injury? Br J Obstet Gynaecol 1985; 92:122–130.

1

The History of the Obstetric Forceps and the Vacuum Extractor

Tis strange—but true; for truth is always strange;
stranger than fiction.
GEORGE GORDON BYRON, 1819
Don Juan
The longer you look back, the further you can look forward.
WINSTON CHURCHILL
March, 1944

History of Obstetric Forceps

Modern obstetric delivery forceps are the modified descendants of various scissor-like, two-bladed destructive instruments dating from antiquity. The history of the development of forceps is colorful and complex and reflects both the inventive genius of many practitioners as well as the influence of their times. The impetus that led to the development of forceps was the observation that a means to assist in obstructed labors was clearly necessary. Before instrumental delivery and cesarean section were possible, fetal destructive procedures or various intrauterine manipulations such as version and extraction were the only techniques available to clinicians when malpresentation or dystocia occurred. Such procedures were often fatal for the fetus and frequently resulted in serious maternal injuries.

Forceps is a word derived from Latin. Literary use of the word forceps goes back at least as far as the writings of Celsus (*De re Medicina*) ca. 50 AD. There are several suggestions for the derivation of the term. "Forceps" may trace its origin to the term *ferricepes*—a contraction of *ferrum*, iron, plus *capio*, "I take," thus, "the iron with

1

which one seizes something hot." Alternatively the word may come from *formus*, "hot," plus *capio*, "I take," thus, "an instrument for picking up something hot."

The origins of forceps for obstetric use are uncertain. Delivery forceps were not known to the Greeks and it is uncertain whether true forceps were used in Roman times. The famous bas-relief from Ostia (ca. 2nd or 3rd century AD) depicting an apparent forceps operation or an instrumental delivery is of uncertain authenticity (1). Certainly there is no extant Roman medical literature describing assisted delivery using instruments designed for saving the fetus. If true obstetric or delivery forceps existed in Roman times, the secret of their use was subsequently lost and did not influence later developments.

Arabic literature including the works of Albucasis, Avicenna, Averoës, and Maimonides dating from 950 to 1200 AD discusses the use of delivery instruments whose name is translated as forceps, but these were devices designed for fetal destruction. For example, the manuscript of Albucasis *On Surgery and Instruments* (2) depicts an instrument with curved, teeth-covered jaws as well as various hooks for obstetrical extractions (Fig. 1.1). Considering their general con-

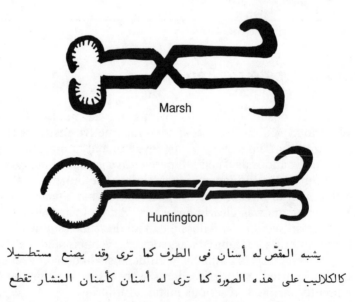

Marsh

Huntington

يشبه المقصّ له أسنان فى الطرف كما ترى وقد يصنع مستطـيلا

كالكلاليب على هذه الصورة كما ترى له أسنان كأسنان المنشار تقطع

Figure 1.1. Destructive delivery instruments described by Albucasis ca. 1000 AD. Illustration depicts portions of the Arabic text and drawings of this instrument in two extant manuscripts (Marsh and Huntington manuscripts, respectively). (From Spink MS, Lewis GL. Albucasis on surgery and instruments. Berkeley, California: University of California Press, 1973.)

struction, these devices must have been designed for postmortem fetal extraction or destruction. No instruments designed for the delivery of a viable or undamaged infant entered European practice from Arabic sources. Prior to the 18th century, European medicine could boast no improvement on this record.

The major European obstetric texts of the 16th and 17th centuries describe instruments designed for assisting obstructed delivery, but again these were for the destruction and removal of the fetus from the uterus rather than for assistance with live births. The work of Eucharius Roesslin (Rösslin), *Der Schwangern Frawen und Hebammen Rosengarten* (1513), largely copied from Soranus' writings (ca. 100 AD) *On Gynecology*, Jacques Rueff's improved Latin version of the same text, *De Conceptu et Generatione Hominis* (1554), Thomas Raynalde's English translation, *The Byrthe of Mankynde* (1552), François Rousset's *Traité Nouveau de l'Hystérotomotokie ou Enfantemente Césarien* (1581), and Scipione Mercurio's *La Comare o Riccoglitrice* (1596) all fail to describe other than destructive or, at the least, highly traumatic instruments (1, 3). Even Ambroise Paré, in his textbook *De la Génération de l'Homme* (1573) in regard to difficult deliveries, says nothing on the use of forceps. As late as 1694 François Mauriceau in the fourth edition of his famous obstetric text, *Traité des Maladies de Femmes Grosses*, mentions only destructive instruments as complements to version and extraction in difficult cases (4).

It was neither technical limitation nor the lack of surgically trained personnel that delayed the development of forceps into the late 17th century. Extraordinary work in steel was the common trade of military armorers throughout the 15th and 16th centuries. Two-bladed articulated metal instruments for obstetric use had been known since the time of Albucasis (ca. 1000 AD). Rueff's 16th century textbook, *De Conceptu et Generatione Hominis* contains illustrations of such instruments (Fig. 1.2), documenting that such devices were in clinical use in Europe before 1560. What was missing was recognition of how to modify and apply this existing technology to the problem of atraumatic delivery. This advance awaited the Chamberlens (5–7).

True delivery forceps were modified from their original destructive purpose to permit relatively atraumatic extraction of a living fetus without inflicting desperate injuries to either mother or child. The design problems for ideal forceps faced obstetric innovators with substantial challenges. It was necessary to fashion an instrument capable of securely grasping the fetal head in order to turn the fetus and/or direct it through the pelvic canal of the mother; however, this assistance needed to be accomplished without serious injury to either passenger or passage.

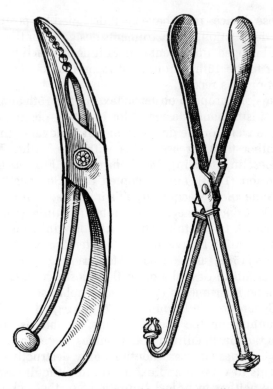

Figure 1.2. Delivery instruments illustrated by Jacques Rueff in *De Conceptu et Generatione Hominis* (1554). (Courtesy of the Historical Division/Cleveland Health Sciences Library, Cleveland, OH.)

Modern forceps are descended from the instruments developed by the Chamberlens, a family of Huguenot refugees who moved to England in the 16th century. William Chamberlen (1540?–1596) fled the St. Bartholomew Day massacres in France and settled in the expatriot French colony in Southampton in 1569. When he died, he left a large family, the majority of whom became physicians and a number of whom, unfortunately for scholars, had the same names (Fig. 1.3). The original William Chamberlen had four sons, two of whom were named Peter. These two sons are commonly referred to as Peter the Younger and Peter the Elder. Peter the Elder, the more successful of the two, had the honor of being called to attend Henrietta Maria, wife of Charles I, in 1628 after the midwife in charge had "swooned with fear" on entering the Queen's chamber. Peter the Elder was probably the inventor of the first forceps. He subsequently passed the secret to his relatives who modified and remodeled the instrument a number of times (Fig. 1.4). This special Chamberlen secret delivery instrument was

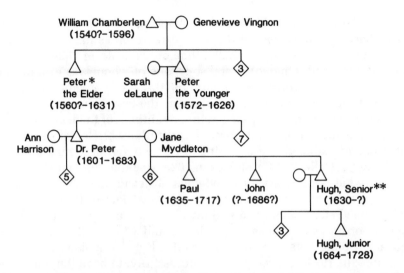

Figure 1.3. Chamberlen family pedigree (5–8, 12). *, Probably the inventor of the Chamberlen forceps; **, Attempted sale of "an instrument" to F. Mauriceau in 1670.

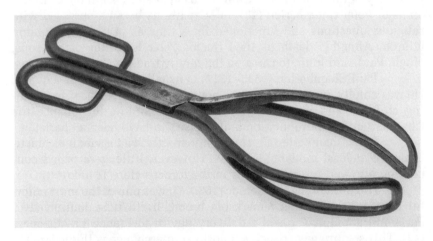

Figure 1.4. Chamberlen delivery forceps ca. 1610 (facsimile). (Courtesy of the Dittrick Museum of Medical History, Historical Division/Cleveland Health Sciences Library, Cleveland, OH.)

transported by two men in a massive, gilt wooden chest. The Chamberlens used a special carriage for its transport so the arrival of "the secret" would be the more spectacular. When the secret was used, other attendants were excluded from the room and the eyes of the laboring woman were blindfolded so even the mother could not later tell exactly what had transpired to achieve delivery (7).

Paradoxically, it was the offspring of the younger Peter Chamberlen who carried on the family tradition, as his older brother apparently left no progeny. By the time of his death in 1626 (8), Peter the Younger had fathered several sons, one of whom was also named Peter. It was this *third* Peter (1601–1683), called "Doctor Peter" because of his university degrees, who was the best trained of the early Chamberlens and the most successful practitioner of them all. He studied in the then prominent medical institutions of Heidelberg, Cambridge, and Padua before returning to London and becoming a fellow of the Royal College of Physicians in 1628. He rapidly established himself in what became a very prestigious obstetric practice in London, serving, among others, members of the royal family (9–11). On his tombstone Peter Chamberlen's family claimed him to have been physician-in-ordinary to James I, Charles I, and Charles II and to their queens. Doctor Peter also became involved in the medical politics of the time. In 1634 he attempted, unsuccessfully, to have the midwives of the city of London incorporated under his control. His distress with this issue led him to publish in 1647 a tract entitled *A Voice in Rhama, or the Cry of the Women and Children as Echoed Forth in the Compassions of Peter Chamberlen* (12). In later life he became obsessed with religious questions and functioned for a time as pastor of a London church. After his death in 1683 Doctor Peter left three of his sons, Hugh, Paul, and John, to carry on the family tradition as obstetricians.

Paul Chamberlen (1635–1717) is usually described as a quack. He was chiefly known for his "celebrated anodyne necklace" for teething children and women in labor. He did nothing to enhance the Chamberlen family reputation and appears to have been a charlatan.

John Chamberlen (?–1686?) apparently was a medical practitioner of at least moderate success. However, little is recorded concerning him and his role, if any, in the forceps story is unknown.

Hugh Chamberlen, Senior (1630–?), was one of the most colorful personalities of this remarkable brood. In 1670 he journeyed to Paris and attempted to sell a delivery device to French practitioners (12). This sojourn gave rise to a notorious interchange with the famous French obstetrician, François Mauriceau (10). Supposedly, Hugh Chamberlen offered to sell the family's secret of delivery to Mauriceau for some 10,000 livres (or thalers?) (13), a vast sum at the time. Chamberlen claimed that his family instrument could deliver even the most difficult of cases. In his recording of this interaction, Mauriceau noted that "... the English doctor spread the report that he had a secret of his own for accouchements of this nature ..." (12). Being no fool and well-versed in the tenets of *caveat emptor*, Mauriceau insisted that "the device" be successfully demonstrated before purchase. Unfortunately for Hugh Chamberlen, the trial case that Mauriceau provided was a dwarf with marked pelvic distortion who had been laboring for a prolonged period of time. Chamberlen aggressively attempted delivery but failed and eventually both the woman and her infant died. At necropsy uterine and genital lacerations were noted. Inevitably, the sale fell through. Not withstanding this debacle Chamberlen maintained friendly relations with Mauriceau and later translated Mauriceau's textbook Traité des Maladies des Femmes Grosses into an English edition that gained rapid popularity. The preface to the second edition of the English translation (1696) contains the only reference to the midwifery forceps ever published by the Chamberlens. In commenting on Mauriceau's use of destructive instruments he stated

I will now take leave to offer an apology for not publishing the secret I have mentioned that we have for extracting children without hooks ... there being my father and two brothers living that practise this art, I cannot esteem it my own to dispose of nor publish it without injury to them, ... the forementioned three persons of our family and myself can serve ... in these extremities with greater safety than others. (From Drinkwater KR. The midwifery forceps: historical sketch. Liverpool Medico-Chirurg J 1913; 64:451–465.)

Some years later in 1693 this same Chamberlen traveled to Holland and apparently sold a delivery device—but possibly not a forceps—to Roger (or Rogier) von Roonhuysen (or van Roonhuyze), a Dutch obstetrician (7, 11, 14). Thereafter the Medical-Pharmacological College of Amsterdam was given the sole privilege of licensing physicians to practice in Holland and required each to purchase "the invention" for a large sum of money under a pledge of complete secrecy. This Dutch connection and its influence on forceps development has always been controversial and unclear. According to Gordon (9) this practice continued for a number of years until Vischer and Van de Poll purchased the secret and made it public. It was then found that the device being sold consisted of a single-bladed instrument (vectis blade?). Dill (14) and Speert (7) relate a somewhat different story. They claim that a practitioner unhappy with this mandatory purchase law (Dr. J. P. Rathlaw?) induced an assistant of von Roonhuysen's, an individual named Van der Swan, to part with a sketch of the secret instrument. The sketch, depicting a set of conventional forceps, was eventually published by Rathlaw in 1747. However, this tale is chronologically suspect as forceps were known in Europe considerably prior to this date. Whether there were two instruments (a vectis blade and forceps) or only one is unclear. In sum, it is possible but not certain that information from Amsterdam originally from the Chamberlens inspired the production of other delivery instruments including Jean Palfyn's *mains de fer* double vectis blade forceps of 1721. Exactly what Chamberlen sold to von Roonhuysen, what, if anything, was communicated to Jean Palfyn in France, or whether the Medical-Pharmacological College of Amsterdam simply swindled the subsequent purchasers of the original secret is not known.

The adventure was not the last for Hugh Chamberlen. In 1690 he hastily left England under suspicion of misappropriation of funds when a scheme for an English land bank failed, although he was apparently not guilty of any wrongdoing (7). He eventually retired to Holland, practicing for some years in Amsterdam prior to his death.

The most prominent son of Hugh Chamberlen was also named Hugh (1664–1728). It was this junior Hugh, also a prominent English obstetrician, who apparently released the family secret about 1720. Hugh Chamberlen, Jr. was educated at Trinity College, Cambridge, graduating with his medical degree in 1689. By 1694 he was a member of the Royal College. An intimate friend of the Duke of Buckingham, he was buried in Westminster Abbey. With the death of Hugh Chamberlen, Jr., the male Chamberlen line was extinguished. However, Chamberlen descendants through the female line are traceable into the 20th century (8).

Obstetric forceps soon came into general use. Alexander Butler of Edinburgh obtained a sample forceps from Dusée in Paris and demonstrated the instrument in 1733 in Scotland (15). By 1733 Edmund Chapman, in his book *A Treatise on the Improvement of Midwifery, Chiefly with Regard to the Operation*, was able to record that forceps were in common use by himself and his colleagues (9, 15). For example, in 1734 Edward Hody published the posthumous *Cases in Midwifery* of William Giffard, a practitioner who died in 1731. Giffard was from Brentwood, approximately 18 miles from Woodham Mortimer, the family home of the Chamberlens. In the case reports are several parturitions in which forceps—called "extractors" in the text—were used for delivery (11). Another practitioner, Benjamin Pugh from Chelmsford, only about 6 miles from Woodham Mortimer, also wrote of his use of forceps before 1750. However, Pugh's work was not published until 4 years later. Thus, it appears that the knowledge of the Chamberlen forceps initially passed locally to several practitioners in a small area of Essex, immediately adjacent to the Chamberlen estate (15). How this was accomplished and who produced these early instruments is unknown.

The final chapter of the Chamberlen story concluded in 1818 when the obstetrical instruments of the Chamberlens were presented to the Royal Medical and Chirurgical Society of London. Peter the Younger's original country home, Woodham Mortimer, had been purchased by a wealthy English brewer. In 1813 the housekeeper found a hidden box under a false floor in a closet. The box contained several obstetrical instruments including four pairs of forceps, presumably representing the progressive modifications and refinements of the original Chamberlen instruments. Also present were levers (vectis blades), crochets, and fillets (6, 9). With the instruments was a document dated 1695, indicating that the box had been concealed following the death of Dr. Peter Chamberlen in 1683.

While the position of the Chamberlens as inventors of forceps appears secure, a possible claimant for independent development of an obstetric delivery instrument is Jean Palfyn (1650–1730) (1, 5). Palfyn, born in Courtrain, Flanders, fabricated a parallel branch forceps or *tire-tête* apparently without direct knowledge of the Chamberlens' device although he may have been influenced indirectly by the Chamberlens' vectis blade (or forceps?) through the Dutch connection as previously suggested. In 1721 at the age of 71, Palfyn went to Paris to demonstrate his *mains de fer* before the French Academy of Sciences. His original model was a double vectis device with blades resembling two large independent spoons, one slightly smaller and more convex than the other, both attached to wooden handles. The response at Palfyn's Paris showing was less than enthusiastic with his critics claiming that his forceps would be impossible to apply in cases of dystocia. Guillaume-Manquest de La Motte (1665–1737), a famous obstetrician of Paris, mentioned in his case commentaries the delivery instrument described by "a certain surgeon of Ghent . . ." (Palfyn) and severely criticized the device as impractical (11). As he wrote (5, 10),

. . . In fact, how could a steel or other instrument pass the place where the head is arrested or incarcerated in such a fashion that we cannot introduce a catheter for the evacuation of urine . . . how, I say, could we introduce this instrument and make it work so precisely that it would draw the child out of the peril to which the narrowness of the canal exposed it? It is certainly a snare and a delusion. If the thing be as TRUE as it is false, and the man die without making this instrument known, he would deserve to have a worm gnaw his entrails throughout eternity, because of the crime he commits in not giving the means of saving the lives of an infinite number of poor children, who perish for want of it, all human science not having been able till now to discover it. But, on the other hand, he will be crowned with benedictions if what he advances be true, for the great good this instrument could do would make him be blessed by God and man. . . . (From Das K. Obstetric forceps: its history and evolution. Calcutta: The Art Press, 1929.)

Following this debacle, Palfyn appears to have become discouraged and he published nothing on the subject of instrumental delivery. Several years later in 1733, Dusée modified Palfyn's original forceps design by crossing the shanks and fitting a screw lock. The blades were also lengthened and the handles flared outward for a better grip. These changes resulted in a much more clinically useful instrument.

It was subsequently claimed that Palfyn did not invent his forceps but copied his idea from the Chamberlens. However, when the prototype forceps of the Chamberlen family were discovered in 1813 they were seen to bear no resemblance to the instrument credited to Palfyn, thus strengthening his claim as an independent inventor (10, 11). The truth of the assertion that Palfyn designed his instrument from plans of a vectis blade obtained from Holland, and thus indirectly from the Chamberlens, will probably never be known.

The inventive genius of the Chamberlens and Palfyn was to develop two-bladed devices without permanently fixed or articulated blades, curving the face of the blade to fit the anatomy of the fetal head (Fig. 1.4.). The unfixed blades permitted easy insertion of the forceps. Chamberlen's blades also were fenestrated, allowing a better grip on the fetal head. The process leading to the development of the Chamberlen forceps is unknown but apparently a workable model had been developed by Peter the Elder about 1610 that was subsequently modified by either him or his descendants. However, as we have seen, the device was kept as a family trade secret until well into the 18th century. Holding back such an important instrument from general use strikes us today as repugnant. However, the Chamberlens were no different in the protection of their own special medical techniques than their contemporaries, and they must be judged by the standards of their own time.

With the emergence of forceps into general obstetric practice after the 1750s, vectis blades also came into increasing prominence although the origin of these instruments is much less clear. A vectis blade is a single metal blade with smooth edges, variably splayed or flattened. One end has some degree of curvature, usually in the distal third of the instrument (16, 17) (Fig. 1.5). Traditionally, the vectis blade is said to have two major purposes: a lever, as in assisting in shoulder dystocia, or as a tractor, with the fenestration hooked over the fetal head or chin (17). The relationship between the development of forceps and the vectis blade is uncertain. It is possible that Hugh Chamberlen in his notorious continental deal may actually have sold a vectis blade to the Medical-Pharmacological College of Amsterdam rather than his best instrument, the forceps. Whether Chamberlen independently invented a vectis instrument, simply sold only a single blade of his forceps, or was peddling an already existing instrument that was then unknown in Holland cannot be determined. It is sometimes stated that Francis Sandes (or Sandys) was the inventor of the

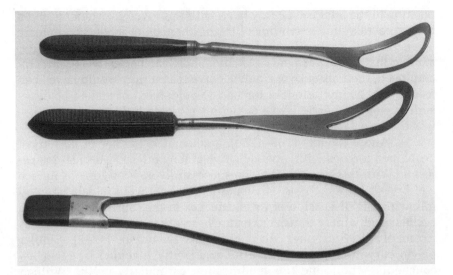

Figure 1.5. Vectis blades and whale bone fillet ca. 1850. (Courtesy of the Dittrick Museum of Medical History, Historical Division/Cleveland Health Sciences Library, Cleveland, OH.)

vectis blade (ca. 1740) but whether he obtained the idea from the Chamberlens or the other way around is also unclear. The primary 19th century proponent of the vectis was Dr. William Lowder who is said to have favored the vectis above forceps, particularly for breech births (16). Whether or not the vectis blade concept was incorporated in the parallel blade forceps of Jean Palfyn is unclear; however, parallel blade instruments apparently inspired by the vectis blade have appeared throughout the history of instrumental delivery. As a single-bladed forceps, such devices are still used to assist cranial extraction at cesarean section (18). An instrument remarkably similar to Palfyn's 18th century model was described as recently as 1960 by Thierry (19). In an article on "the toboggan maneuver" a double vectis instrument for vaginal delivery was presented that appears to be a modern counterpart of the Palfyn device. More practical designs incorporating the same idea include the modern divergent blade forceps of Laufe and the parallel blade instrument of Shute (20).

Both the Palfyn and various Chamberlen forceps were far from ideal. They were short, straight instruments with only a cephalic curve. The Chamberlen models were all fenestrated and apparently all could be (or were) articulated. Further, in most instances, applications with these early instruments were pelvic and not cephalic; that is, the blades were applied in the same fashion to all cases, regardless of the position of the fetal head. Only later, with improved instruments and a better practical understanding of the mechanism of labor did cephalic or anatomically specific applications become standard practice. Assuming that the instruments of Palfyn and Chamberlen were correctly employed, their absence of a pelvic curve meant they would have been useful only as low or outlet forceps. Development of angled blades— addition of the pelvic curve to permit more complex applications— was the next major innovation in forceps design.

André Levret (1703–1780), a celebrated teacher of obstetrics, developed forceps with a pelvic curve among other obstetrical instruments. With this modification, he successfully applied forceps in face and breech presentations. His modified forceps were widely adapted following his discussion of its advantages in the fourth edition of his popular and widely translated text, *Observations sur les Causes et les Accidents de Plusieures Accouchements Laborieux* (1747). Similar pelvic curve instruments were independently invented by other accoucheurs, who found this modification particularly useful. William Smellie between 1745 and 1753, described the use of an instrument incorporating a pelvic curve. Benjamin Pugh apparently developed the same idea, writing in 1754 of "the forceps I invented upward of 14 years ago" incorporating this innovation (3). The addition of the pelvic curve helped accommodate the forceps to the shape of the birth canal, permitting a more accurate, less traumatic application. In what proved to be a mixed blessing this design modification led to higher extractions and soon, rotational deliveries with the associated increased maternal/fetal risk in poorly trained hands.

William Smellie (1697–1763), born in Lanark, Scotland, was the most prominent British practitioner of the 18th century (3, 21). He was one of the first obstetricians to study and teach the use of forceps although he employed the instrument with great discretion. He was also a careful student of pelvic anatomy and invented the perforating delivery scissors that still bear his name. When called to attend a delivery, he concealed his forceps from onlookers and patient alike, an easy feat in his time when the obstetrician wore a long coat with deep pockets that served to hide the instruments. Such concealment was necessary. So great was the prejudice against the use of forceps in Smellie's time that it was possible to apply them only without the knowledge of either the midwife or the patient. Smellie covered the metal blades of his forceps with wrappings of thin leather, not only to take away the chill and achieve a better hold but also to spare the patient the sound of clicking metal as the blades were articulated (9, 11). This may also have reduced the patient's recognition that she was being instrumented for delivery. Smellie did note the importance of changing the leather if he suspected the person on whom the forceps were used of having a venereal infection (22). His text, *Anatomic Tables* (1754), was an important contribution to obstetric literature, notable for its anatomically accurate and beautiful illustrations (Fig. 1.6).

Influential contemporaries of Smellie were strongly opposed to forceps use. William Hunter (1718–1783), a pupil of Smellie, practiced obstetrics much more conservatively. Hunter was not only a leading London obstetrician, but he also made a place in medical history with his exquisite atlas, *The Anatomy of the Human Gravid Uterus* (1774) (23). He was also notable for his anatomic research and collections. His accumulated anatomic and other specimens, along with the collection of Dr. John Fothergill, now form the basis of the Hunterian Museum of Glasgow (9, 23, 24). In his obstetric practice Hunter allowed nature to take its course whenever possible. He rarely used forceps. In fact, he was wont to publicly exhibit his own rusty pair during obstetric lectures as proof of this fact.

The safe and effective application of forceps was advanced by the Danish obstetrician Matthias Saxtorph (1740–1800), a noted master of clinical medicine and a student of the mechanism of labor. He was among the first to demonstrate the importance of traction in the pelvic axis. In 1772 he proposed a combined two-handed traction technique for instrumental delivery later described by Osiander and Charles P. Pajot and now commonly termed the Saxtorph-Pajot maneuver.

Obstetrics, along with medicine in general, underwent revolutionary changes in the 19th century, resulting in the rapid development of new techniques and procedures. Use of these new aids for therapy and diagnosis began hesitantly in the opening years but after the midcentury, along with the general enthusiasm of society for invention and innovation, physician interest in mechanical contrivances in medicine accelerated. Technology appeared to offer new means to combat dystocia, avoid fetal-maternal injury, and apply scientific principles to what previously was held to be largely an art. However, these changes came neither easily nor without controversy.

Uncritical and often faulty use of obstetric instrumentation had followed the introduction of forceps in the mid-18th century. Inevitably, a school of cautionary practice developed among major practitioners of obstetrics, principally in England, in reaction to these excesses (25). William Hunter and Thomas Denmon (1733–1815) were among the most notable proponents of "leaving to nature." These practitioners and their followers would not intervene with operative delivery except under extreme conditions and then only following mark-

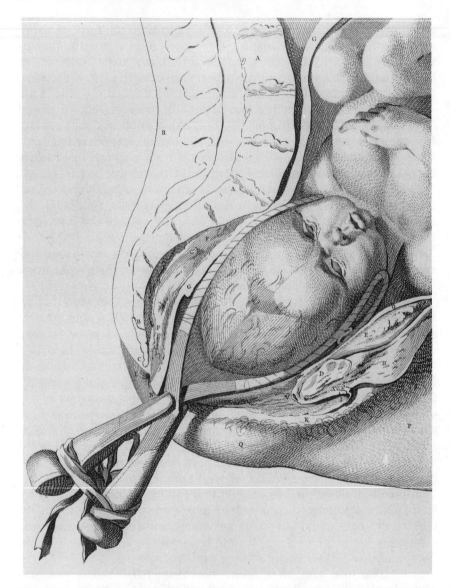

Figure 1.6.   Smellie forceps applied to the left occiput transverse as depicted in his text, *Anatomical Tables* (1754) (22). (Courtesy of the Historical Division/Cleveland Health Sciences Library, Cleveland, OH.)

edly prolonged labor. The unreality of this approach was exposed in 1818 in the tragic delivery of Princess Charlotte, only daughter of the Prince Regent of England (25–28). The attending physician, Dr. Richard Croft, permitted the Princess to labor after full dilatation for more than 24 hours. Tragically both the infant and the mother died. Three months later Dr. Croft committed suicide in despondency, unable to bear the criticism of his management. The result, a ". . . mother, baby, accoucheur, all dead, all victims most likely of a mistaken system, a bad patch, a veritable craze of midwifery practice . . ." (27). The extreme view against any instrumentation as championed by Denman (Croft's father-in-law) paved the way to this disaster. The childbirth death of Princess Charlotte provoked serious social and political problems by destroying two generations of heirs to the British throne. At the time there was not a single legitimate heir from the offspring of George III and Queen Charlotte. Without a legitimate heir the crown would pass to the Duke of Brunswick, a cousin of George III, living in Hanover—an event hardly likely to be well received in England. The three most likely princes, the Duke of Clarence, the Duke of Kent, and the Duke of Cambridge, although of middle age and despite various prior attachments, set to the task of attempting to produce an acceptable (i.e., legitimate) heir for the throne. This eventually led in 1819 to the delivery of Victoria, who ascended the throne in 1837 for what proved to be the longest continuous rule of any English monarch.

Obstetric events and the use of instrumentation also influenced history on the continent of Europe. Antoine Dubois (1756–1839) performed a successful forceps operation in 1811 on Marie-Louise, wife of Napoleon Bonaparte, that had international repercussions (1). Napoleon's son was macrosomic and the aftercoming head was entrapped. This "dystocie de la tête dernière" was overcome by a forceps application. With active resuscitation by Dubois, the infant boy, fated to be (temporarily) the King of Rome, survived. This delivery eventually brought Dubois the title of baron and 100,000 francs, delight to Napoleon, and distress to Italy (1, 29).

In the latter half of the 19th century, a virtual revolution in medical and surgical therapeutics accompanied rapid advances in the understanding of the mechanisms of disease. The advent of anesthesia in the mid-1840s and the development of the germ theory in the 1860s reinforced the ties between medicine and technology (30–32). Suddenly the pathophysiology of previously mysterious disorders was explicable and physicians began to believe that they could improve upon nature. New technical information modified obstetric practice in complex ways. For example, the introduction of anesthetics in the form of ether, nitrous oxide, and chloroform rendered patients unconscious or insensible to pain, thus allowing greater latitude for surgical intervention and increased time to achieve results (31). The development of antisepsis in the 1860s and asepsis in the 1880s reduced the morbidity of surgical intervention. As the possibilities of increasingly favorable outcome developed, more women were inclined to accept surgical procedures for delivery as salvation for themselves and their infants. Not surprisingly, new operations and procedures soon followed (5, 33). However, due to lack of clear standards, an absence of effective regulatory bodies, multiple practitioners of doubtful competence, and a *laissez faire* attitude toward human experimentation, the return of uncontrolled instrumentation took a toll in maternal and fetal injury.

From 1860 onward substantial changes in obstetrical instrumentation occurred (5, 30, 33). Physicians who were adherents of Joseph Lister believed that disinfectants, chiefly carbolic acid or phenol, or boiling would render instruments germ free and hence safe. Instruments with handles of bone, ebony, and various woods suffered adversely from this treatment so these materials were soon replaced by hard rubber called vulcanite (in America) and ebonite (in Britain). Once cleansed by Listerian techniques, instruments were carefully dried and replaced in lined wooden boxes or rolled in cloth pocket cases (Fig. 1.7). Yet, by the late 1880s it was clear that traditional instrument design, construction, and materials precluded complete sterilization. Samples of ostensibly sterile instruments revealed that bacterial contamination was rampant despite standard antiseptic precautions, and new techniques were needed (34).

The new demands of asepsis and steam sterilization forced fundamental changes in the design and construction of medical instruments. Handle materials and construction methods needed modification. Thus, cracks and crevices in instruments that precluded cleaning were progressively removed. Hard rubber, fabric, and wooden parts disappeared giving way to instruments fabricated entirely of chromed or forged stainless steel and capable of resisting the heat and pressure of the new techniques of steam sterilization. The previously popular, highly polished cast steel instruments with carefully fitted checkered ebony handles were supplanted by one-piece alloy steel instruments devoid of ornamentation (Fig. 1.8). Beauty and quality of instruments would henceforth be defined strictly in terms of functionality and simplicity, virtues forced by technical innovation (30).

Several obstetricians left their mark in obstetric history during these exciting and turbulent times. James Young Simpson (1811–1870) developed not only a type of forceps but also the first effective obstetric vacuum extractor. Simpson was a socially active, highly regarded teacher and clinician and an influential obstetric leader in England. He introduced forceps of his special design in 1848. This instrument rapidly became popular and is in common use today (see Figs. 2.1 and 2.2). Simpson authored papers on hospital design, mesmerism, acupressure, and homeopathy among other subjects. He was strongly

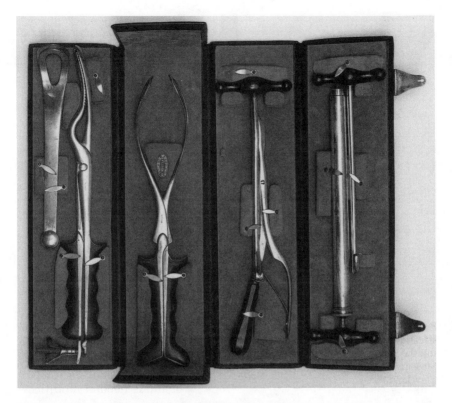

Figure 1.7.   A presentation case of obstetrical instruments ca. 1870. Note the presence of vectis blades (*left*) and several destructive instruments in addition to the regular forceps. (Courtesy of the Dittrick Museum of Medical History, Historical Division/Cleveland Health Sciences Library, Cleveland, OH.)

interested in archaeology. In addition, he played a pivotal role in developing obstetric anesthesia. Following experiments upon himself and his colleagues he discovered the anesthetic properties of chloroform and described its use during delivery as well as in the treatment of eclamptic seizures (35, 36). Simpson successfully defended chloroform against his antagonists who opposed its use in obstetrics on moral grounds. In 1853, chloroform was administered to Queen Victoria for the delivery of her eighth pregnancy. Following a discussion with her doctors concerning the proposed and controversial use of this anesthetic, the queen remarked, "Gentlemen, We are having the baby and We are having the chloroform. . . ." This event strongly influenced the subsequent general acceptance of obstetric anesthesia (37).

George T. Elliott (1827–1871), a New York City native, invented his "new midwifery forceps" 10 years after Simpson described

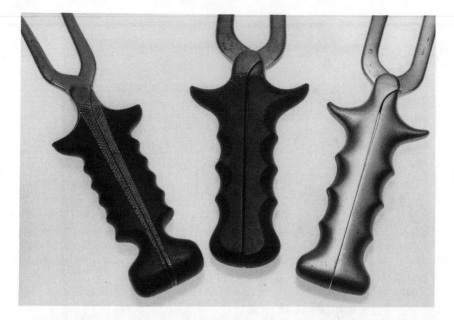

Figure 1.8. Late 19th century Simpson design forceps. Note changes in handle construction and decoration from left to right—ebony to hard rubber to all metal—paralleling the introduction of aseptic techniques for sterilization. (Courtesy of the Dittrick Museum of Medical History, Historical Division/Cleveland Health Sciences Library, Cleveland, OH.)

his instrument. Elliot's specific intention was to avoid undue compression of the fetal head. Thus, he designed a set screw in the handle of his instrument to regulate the degree to which the blades could be approximated—an idea probably originated by J. Aitken in 1794 (14). Along with Simpson's forceps, Elliot's are the most popular of the classic forceps (see Figs. 2.1 and 2.2). Educated at Columbus College and receiving his medical degree from the University of New York, Elliot studied in Europe for 3 years prior to his appointment to the staff of Bellevue Hospital (38). From 1861 until his early death at the age of 44 he was Professor of Obstetrics and Diseases of Women and Children at the Bellevue Hospital Medical College. He was a noted lecturer and did not restrict his medical interests to obstetrics. His principal work, *Obstetric Clinic*, was published in 1868.

Other obstetric innovators were also at work and the bewildering assortment of their instruments fills page after page of Das' monumental monograph on forceps (5). Robert Barnes (1817–1907) designed a set of forceps to enable delivery from the superior strait and from above the brim in cephalopelvic disproportion. His aim was to reduce the incidence of craniotomy. He designed a unique instrument with a long, relatively flat cephalic curve to fit the greatly molded fetal head formed after days of labor. The extra length in the shank and blades turned out to be unnecessary, however, because it only increased maternal discomfort and the risk of soft tissue damage (39).

Hugh Lenox Hodge (1796–1873) was a champion of proper indications for forceps use. Trained at Princeton and the University of Pennsylvania, he became a highly regarded teacher of obstetrics and gynecology. His forceps (Fig. 1.9) featuring a marked cephalic curve were modified from the instruments of André Levret (1747) and Louis A. Baudelocque (1781), following classic French style. His text, *The Principles and Practice of Obstetrics* (1864), was influential in the 19th century practice of obstetrics. For many years Professor of Obstetrics and Diseases of Women and Children at the University of Pennsylvania (1835–1863), he anticipated the Credé method of placental expulsion and wrote on the mechanism of labor. In modern practice, his name is primarily recalled because of his pessary for uterine displacement. In practice he crusaded against induced abortion and opposed *accouchement forcé* in eclamptic patients. Less happily he was also a vocal critic of the concept of the contagiousness of puerperal septicemia (40).

In the latter portion of the 19th century great interest in the mechanism of labor developed, prompted in part by the earlier work of Saxtorph. Before long these ideas were reflected in the design of new delivery instruments. A new principle in forceps construction, the

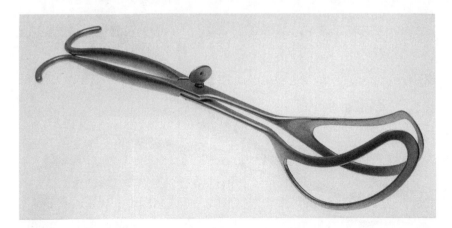

Figure 1.9. Hodge forceps ca. 1833 (5). Note French lock, hooks at handle ends, parallel shanks, and tight cephalic curve. (Courtesy of the Dittrick Museum of Medical History, Historical Division/Cleveland Health Sciences Library, Cleveland, OH.)

compensation curve, was introduced in 1860 by L. J. Hubert. In this design, Hubert bent the forceps handles backward at right angles, allowing traction in a direct line with the pelvic curve. This permitted a more accurate alignment of the fetal head through the birth canal and less force exerted on the head. Hubert's design was a forerunner of the axis traction forceps of Etienne Stephene Tarnier (1828–1897) (5). Tarnier was a major contributor to obstetrical knowledge. He was interested in contagiousness of puerperal infection and confirmed the ideas initially brought forth by I. P. Semmelweis. In 1877 after exhaustive experimentation and modification, Tarnier presented to the French Academy of Medicine his traction forceps (Fig. 1.10). The success of these forceps spawned a plethora of similar instruments. The virtues of axis traction were loudly proclaimed by Charles P. Pajot (1816–1896). An energetic and aggressive teacher of obstetrics for nearly half a century, Pajot was renowned for his anecdotes and aphorisms and was virtually unrivalled in France as a clinical practitioner (1, 5, 41–44).

Other practitioners refined axis traction. In 1891 Robert Milne Murray described a forceps and axis traction handle designed "to draw the foetal head through the pelvic canal with the least expenditure of force."

Solid-bladed forceps, originally described by Osiander in 1799, were reintroduced by Malcolm McLane in the 1880s to make rotations easier (14). Later in the 20th century R. Luikart (45) modified

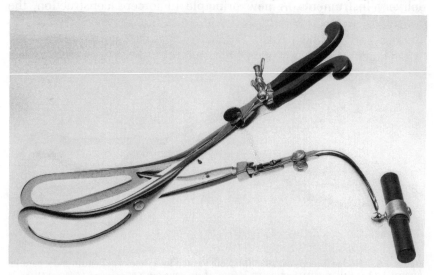

Figure 1.10. Tarnier axis traction forceps ca. 1880. (Courtesy of the Dittrick Museum of Medical History, Historical Division/Cleveland Health Sciences Library, Cleveland, OH.)

the nonfenestrated blades by thinning the interior portion while leaving the edges thicker, an idea apparently dating back to A. Hohl in 1850 (14). This pseudofenestration reduced the chances of fetal injury but maintained a firm grip on the fetal head (Fig. 1.11).

The master of rotational deliveries was Friedrich Wilhelm Scanzoni (1821–1891). Scanzoni worked in Prague, the city of his birth, as well as in Wurtzburg. He is most noted for his grand rotation for the occiput posterior presentation, introduced in 1851. Similar techniques were known earlier to Smellie and probably to others, but to Scanzoni goes the credit for popularizing the procedure. The Scanzoni maneuver is a complete 180° instrumental rotation performed by rotating the fetal head from occiput posterior position to occiput anterior or oblique position with a second application for outlet delivery (20, 46). Modified in various fashions, this maneuver is still performed (14, 20, 47).

Arthur Holbrook Bill, M.D. (1877–1961) of the Western Reserve University School of Medicine in Cleveland developed a new axis traction handle which permitted excellent traction and the use of standard forceps (48). His device consisted of a metal cage that fitted over the lock and shanks of a classic obstetric forceps. An articulated handle was fitted including an indicator which pointed in the direction of traction (Fig. 1.11). Occasionally this axis traction device is still used clinically.

Other clinicians modified forceps for specific clinical indications. Lyman Guy Barton (1866–1944) developed a unique forceps for transverse arrests (Fig. 2.13) (49, 50). Barton was trained at Dartmouth College and Bellevue Hospital Medical School, graduating in 1891. After graduation he assumed the responsibility for his father's prac-

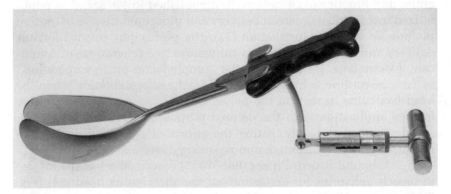

Figure 1.11. Bill's axis traction handle with spring loaded force indicator applied to Tucker-McLane forceps (48). (Courtesy of the Dittrick Museum of Medical History, Historical Division/Cleveland Health Sciences Library, Cleveland, OH.)

tice. Throughout his career his original training in mechanical engineering was of assistance. Barton designed a number of medical instruments including obstetric forceps. During World War I he acted as a radiologist due to the temporary absence of the radiologist on active military service. By 1932 he was asked to take charge of the x-ray department at Physicians' Hospital in Plattsburgh, NY, a city to which he had moved in 1914 following his progressive involvement with more extensive surgical procedures. Barton's forceps were an answer to the problem of the handling of the fetal head in transverse arrest (20, 47, 50).

Christian Kielland (1871–1941) also developed forceps for use in midpelvic arrest. Kielland, working in Oslo, introduced his design in 1915 (51) (Fig. 2.12). Kielland's forceps are unique among more modern designs for their virtually absent pelvic curve and use of a sliding lock. Kielland's instrument was designed primarily for midpelvic rotations and thus did not need to accommodate to the shape of the birth canal. These forceps also proved useful in the rotation of occiput posterior positions and historically in the delivery of face presentations. The sliding lock was specifically added to permit correction of the asynclitism common in transverse midpelvic arrest.

Joseph Bolivar DeLee (1869–1942) made a prominent mark in 20th century obstetric practice in the United States. Graduating from Chicago Medical College in 1891 he established the Chicago Lying-In Dispensary in 1895 that subsequently became the Chicago Lying-In Hospital that merged with the University of Chicago (52). He held the rank of Professor of Obstetrics at Northwestern University for nearly 40 years. He designed delivery equipment, forceps, and a stethoscope during his long career. His most important work was his text *The Principles and Practice of Obstetrics*, first published in 1913. DeLee popularized low cervical cesarean delivery and pioneered the use of motion pictures in obstetric instruction (52). His philosophy toward forceps delivery and episiotomy strongly influenced two generations of American obstetricians. He described the "prophylactic forceps operation" as ". . . the routine delivery of the child in head presentation when the head has come to rest on the pelvic floor. . . ." He proposed routine forceps application with the defined purpose of ". . . relieving pain, supplementing and anticipating the efforts of Nature, reducing the hemorrhage, and preventing and repairing damages" (53).

Edmund Brown Piper (1881–1935) described a forceps for use in breech deliveries for extractions of the aftercoming head (54) (Fig. 2.14). Born in Williamsport, PA, he first entered a business career following graduation from Princeton (52). Five years later he entered medical school and after graduation was swept up in World War I where he commanded several camp hospitals. After the war, he resumed practice in Philadelphia, becoming Professor of Obstetrics and Gynecology at the University of Pennsylvania. His forceps, described following 5 years of development, were specialized for assisting breech delivery and have never been surpassed for this application.

History of the Ventouse or the Vacuum Extractor

The development of a vacuum instrument for delivery—the obstetric vacuum extractor or ventouse as it is known in European literature—had its origin in the ancient technique of cupping. Initially, several medical innovators applied the cupping principle in devising suction devices to treat depressed skull fracture and to assist at obstetric delivery. However, vacuum extraction for obstetric purposes remained an obscure technique until James Young Simpson championed his "suction tractor" in 1849. After a brief flurry of interest sparked by Simpson's writing, the vacuum extractor essentially disappeared from the obstetric literature except for an occasional paper or vocal proponent until the mid-20th century. Today, especially in Europe, vacuum extraction has essentially replaced the forceps as the primary method of assisted delivery. For interested readers, the history of the obstetric vacuum extraction is reviewed in detail by Chalmers (55, 56), Sjöstedt (57), Malmström (58, 59), and Thiery (60).

In 1632, Hildanus (61) first reported the use of the vacuum for traction on body parts when he treated depressed skull fractures in infants with a leather sucker. The prominent French surgeon Ambroise Paré also described applying a cupping glass to a depressed fracture of the skull. Of interest, Paré indicated the importance of patient assistance in the procedure. As he described, "if the bones do not spring back of themselves, you must apply a cupping glass with a great flame, . . . with all commanding the patient [to] force [his] breath up as powerfully as he can, keeping his mouth and nose shut." A similar technique using a hand breast pump has recently proven successful in elevation of the depressed "ping pong ball" skull fractures of newborns.

The history of the earliest applications of vacuum to assist delivery is lost. There are, however, data indicating that vacuum extraction was practiced well before its mid-19th century rediscovery. In 1694, James Younge (1646–1721), surgeon to the naval hospital at Plymouth and mayor of that city, recorded in his case notes an instance of prolonged labor in which a vacuum device was applied. He reported he was "call to deliver . . . a woman four days in labour . . ." but could neither "fasten the crotchet nor draw it out by a cupping glass fixt to the scalp with an air pump . . . in this extremity, I directed my son to open the child's head. This was soon and easily done and delivery completed" (63).

Little more was heard of vacuum extraction as an obstetric delivery technique until James Young Simpson announced the development of his "suction tractor." Because of his prestige, experience, and successful use of his vacuum device, Simpson is generally given the credit as the inventor of the first practical obstetric vacuum extractor (35, 55, 64).

The idea for a vacuum-based instrument to assist in deliveries apparently occurred to Simpson as early as the mid-1830s. Robert Patterson in a letter of 7 April 1849 recalled how he and Simpson "passing along the street together in 1836 . . . happened to come upon a group of boys lifting large stones with round pieces of wetted leather commonly called suckers." Later references by Simpson reveal that he was also aware of the prior proposals of Neil Arnott as well as the works of Ambroise Paré and Hildanus (55, 64). It is presumed that from the proposals of his predecessors and his own experience Simpson developed the idea for a vacuum-operated device for obstetric use.

Simpson announced his vacuum device in 1849 (35). Apparently, he developed a first model by fitting a metal vaginal speculum with a vacuum piston. The trumpet shaped end of this device was covered with pliable leather which was greased with lard prior to application. When the piston was evacuated, vacuum was produced, securing the instrument to the fetal scalp. Thereafter traction was applied to the body of the instrument for delivery. Progressively modifying his extractor, Simpson subsequently described a more effective model consisting of a cup of "vulcanised caoutchouc" and an attached "double valve piston" pump. This device was remarkably similar in function and appearance to contemporary 19th century and even some currently available models of breast pumps. Whether breast pump design or technology influenced Simpson in the execution of his various models is unknown. In his last "improved model," Simpson added a brass wire diaphragm within the hollow of the cup to prevent fetal scalp injury when vacuum was produced. Simpson reported that with the new device and a good application ". . . I lifted . . . an iron weight of 26 lbs. It could lift double . . ." (56). An example of Simpson's air tractor is still preserved at the Department of Obstetrics and Gynecology at the University of Edinburgh (Fig. 1.12).

The deciding factor for Simpson in construction of his traction instrument may have been his observation of "the artificial French

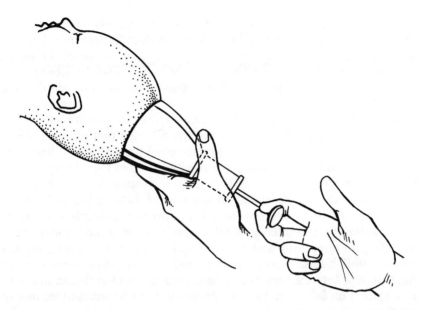

Figure 1.12.   Simpson's "air tractor" vacuum extractor, 1849. (Modified from Thiery M. Obstetric vacuum extraction. Obstet Gynecol Annu 1985; 14:73–111.

leech," a device devised by Guidicelli in 1847 that incorporated suction in an apparatus designed for blood letting (65). Simpson recorded that he had thought and talked of making a "tractor" for years but "in December, 1848, after observing the artificial French leech, I thought that an exhausting cylinder on the same principle would answer the purpose" (55). Simpson clearly used his device clinically. He reported that he had "... employed it repeatedly in both cephalic and pelvic presentations and both when the head was already high above the brim and already sunk deep into the pelvic cavity..." (56).

Contemporaries of Simpson were also involved in experimentation or speculation concerning obstetric vacuum extraction. John Haddy James (1788–1869) described a vacuum cup with suction produced by an attached syringe. He proposed that such an instrument could be used in cases of uterine inertia or dystocia, especially when the fetal head was too high to permit the easy use of the forceps. He also stated that the device could promote delivery of retained placentae. He apparently never constructed such an instrument but discussed the idea for the device in the same issue of the London Medical Gazette in which Simpson's original paper was published.

Neil Arnott (1788–1874) was another medical personality who became involved in promoting the technique of vacuum extraction. Originally trained as a surgeon, he entered the East India Company where, among other adventures, he undertook several voyages to China. In 1827, Arnott published a book entitled *Elements of Physics or Natural Philosophy* in which he advocated the use of an air or "pneumatic tractor" to assist delivery (66). It is unclear whether an instrument such as he described ever existed; however, he did discuss the design of such a device. He suggested a cup be constructed of circular leather or other soft substance, extended by solid rings. Such a tractor, he commented, "seems peculiarly adapted to a purpose of obstetrical surgery, viz., as a substitute for steel forceps in the hands of men who are deficient in manual dexterity, whether from inexperience or natural ineptitude." In addition, Arnott proposed that his tractor might "assist in raising depressed portions of fractured skull" (56).

Surprisingly, despite the initial apparent successes of Simpson's tractor and the interest of other practitioners, vacuum extraction failed to gain popularity and soon lapsed into obscurity. Even Simpson did not publish further on vacuum extraction after 1849. Thus, despite this flurry of interest and innovation, after the mid-19th century vacuum extraction fell from the mainstream of obstetric thought for nearly 100 years, except for an occasional vocal proponent.

In the remaining years of the 19th century, other vacuum-operated devices for achieving delivery were described by Soubhy Saleh (1857), Herbert L. Stillman (1875), and P. McCahey (1890) (56). The latter described several types of "atmospheric tractors." In these devices, a vacuum pump was separated from the cup and traction mechanism. McCahey's most successful cup was soft rubber with which he reported successful accouchement in five cases. Kuntzsch of Potsdam (1912) described a "vakuum helm" consisting of a metal reinforced rubber cup attached to a vacuum pump with a pressure gauge. A further series of various vacuum devices were described during the 1930s and 1940s but none of these became popular. For example, R. Torpin in 1939 described a suction cup device, apparently developed from a sectioned rubber ball, that was reported to have been successfully applied in 13 cases (56). He claimed that his instrument was also useful in rotation of the fetal head.

The most clinically successful ventouse before invention of the Malmström instrument was a device devised by V. Finderle in the early 1950s. This extractor used an elongated conically shaped cup fitted with a flexible rubber cuff on the end applied to the fetal scalp. Vacuum was provided by a syringe. By 1961 Finderle had reported successful applications in 220 deliveries (56). Despite these apparent clinical successes, Finderle's apparatus never achieved popularity.

What eventually proved to be the most successful vacuum extractor was described by T. Malmström of Gothenburg, Sweden, in

1953, with an improved version following in 1956 (58, 67). Malmström's original intention was to design a vacuum device to pull the fetal head against the cervix presumably improving and accelerating the progress of labor in the first stage in instances of uterine inertia (56). This principle is similar to that proposed by Willett in 1925 (68) with his scalp traction forceps. This original idea—to use a vacuum device to assist in the first stage of labor—never gained acceptability in American practice but did attract European adherents. Subsequently the Malmström vacuum extractor became used as a substitute for forceps, with many of the same indications.

Malmström's device was successful and incorporates several features developed by his predecessors and included in earlier instruments. The cup, made of metal, is available in various sizes and contains an internal plastic or metal protective disc, as originally suggested by Simpson, to avoid drawing the fetal scalp into the suction port. The vacuum cup is connected by flexible rubber or plastic tubing to a vacuum source with a glass collecting bottle positioned between the two, similar to the design of McCahey. Finally, the Malmström system, like that of Kuntzsch, incorporates a pressure gauge to judge the strength of vacuum (56).

Following Malmström's a number of other vacuum extractors have been described. A partial listing is given in Table 1.1. The major-

Table 1.1.   Modified Vacuum Extractors

Author	Description
I. Devices Modified for Oblique Traction	
Lovset (69)	Metal cup with four lateral traction cords
Party (70)	Plastic cup with flexible traction stalk
Saling and Rothe (71)	Metal cup with rigid handle attached by ball and socket joint
O'Neil et al. (72)	Metal cup with rotating traction collar
Bird (73)	Metal Malmström-design "OP" cup with laterally attached suction port and nylon cord traction at cup edge
II. Devices Employing Modified Cup Design	
Halkin (74)	Metal Malmström-design cup with reduced height
Sjöstedt (57)	Metal cup with flattened center and shortened suction tube
Bird (75)	Metal Malmström-design cup with suction port separated from central traction site
III. Devices with Flexible Cup Design	
Pelosi and Apuzzio (76)	Funnel-shaped silastic cup with metal traction/vacuum valve handle (Kobayashi device)
Wood (77) and Paul et al. (78)	Polyethylene disposable device with semirigid plastic cup with attached handle

ity of these devices were developed as modifications of Malmström's original design. Various changes were introduced to reduce the likelihood of cup detachment, facilitate application, or better protect the fetal scalp.

Bird's modification (75) has proven the most convenient and popular. In Bird's design, the vacuum tube is attached to a lateral suction port independent of the attachment of the traction chain. A detachable traction handle hooks onto the traction chain at any convenient position once the cup is in place. Bird's cup is much easier to assemble than Malmström's original instrument and has virtually replaced it in clinical use. Unfortunately, the Malmström extractor with Bird's modification is not presently available in the United States due to problems in product liability insurance. Whether this unfortunate state of affairs is permanent is uncertain. However, large numbers of Malmström type extractors, predominately of Bird's modified design, still survive in the obstetric armamentarium of clinical services.

Two other recently developed instruments are still commercially available; a flexible instrument produced from silastic plastic originally designed by Kobayashi (76) and a semirigid polyethylene disposable device (77, 78). Both of these instruments come in a single cup size only.

The eventual acceptance and popularization of vacuum extraction was due both to changing ideas about the appropriateness of obstetric interference as well as technical advances permitting the construction of certain devices. Vacuum extraction had its origin in cupping—the ancient technique of extracting blood or other fluids by evacuating a glass or metal dome and applying it to a patient's skin (60). Blood letting by such methods was a common practice in the 18th and 19th centuries. Such techniques would have been familiar to Simpson and his contemporaries who first seriously attempted to develop vacuum extractors. It had long been clear that cupping developed considerable negative pressure as long as a good seal could be maintained to the patient's skin. The basis of the vacuum technique in obstetric delivery, that is, applying force to the fetal scalp for delivery, depended upon combining the technique of cupping with a means to generate sufficient vacuum on demand. The traditional method for cupping—heating a glass or metal cup with an open flame before application—obviously presented problems for obstetric use. Further, acceptable methods of maintaining a firm seal to the fetal scalp and applying traction to the cup once it was attached had to be developed. By the time Simpson conceived his extractor in 1849, several technical advances had occurred to assure its success. Flexible substances such as vulcanized rubber were available for cup margins, and instrument makers had developed vacuum syringes machined to close tolerances capable of producing powerful suction. Also, medical innovations were common at the time with many new techniques and devices entering obstetric practice easing the acceptance of novel procedures. Finally, Simpson was a most influential practitioner and his championing of any technique guaranteed an attentive audience.

Judging from his clinical descriptions, Simpson apparently used his instrument in the second stage of labor as an alternative to forceps. Considering the design of his tractor, some applications must have been difficult, limited by the relative length and inflexibility of the instrument and problems of maintaining a seal. The vacuum syringe system was attached permanently to the suction cup which must have interfered with maintenance of adequate vacuum due to imperfections in the seal. Any significant leakage would have required reapplication of the cup. Also, in the operation of the device, the accoucheur was required to use both hands actively at once, one to grasp the body of the instrument for traction while the other maintained the syringe plunger at full extension to retain suction. This must have been a clumsy arrangement at best. In comparison, the forceps available at the time were superior instruments. Due to these technical limitations, it is not surprising that Simpson's interest in vacuum extraction waned and that such devices did not become popular until these technical problems were solved.

The resurrection of vacuum extraction in the late 1950s and 1960s was due to a combination of factors. European obstetric practice is more heavily dependent upon midwifery and other nonphysician attendants than is true in the United States. The extensive training necessary for traditional instrumental delivery and the maternal trauma possible with forceps applications was well-recognized. Thus, an instrument less traumatic than forceps but capable of assisting delivery, especially if usable by lesser trained personnel and possible to use with local anesthesia, found a ready market. The development of effective vacuum pumps capable of automatically maintaining a constant preset negative pressure, improved metal suctions cups, and the introduction of flexible plastics provided the final technical innovations necessary for the development of the modern extractor.

Thus, modern practitioners have the inheritance of a rich past. From the first crude instruments of the Chamberlens to the divergent blades of Laufe and the silastic vacuum extractor, literally hundreds of operative delivery instruments have been described (5, 10, 14, 20, 47, 79). Modifications were made to answer a particular clinical problem or for operator convenience. The major events in the history of instrumental delivery are worth emphasis (Table 1.2). Practitioners of the art

Table 1.2. Major Events in the History of Instrumental Delivery

First practical forceps including a cephalic curve and atraumatic blades	H. Chamberlen, ca. 1610 (?)
Invention of pelvic curve	A. Levret, 1747
	W. Smellie, ca. 1750
	B. Pugh, ca. 1740
Development of the technique of rotational delivery	W. Smellie, ca 1745–1750
Invention of the English lock	W. Smellie, 1752
Invention of a practical vacuum extractor	J. Simpson, 1849
Discovery of anesthesia	
Ether	C. W. Long, 1842
	T. G. Morton, 1846
Chloroform	J. Simpson, 1847
Development of axis traction	L. J. Hubert, 1860
	E. S. Tarnier, 1877
Introduction of "prophylactic forceps delivery"	J. B. DeLee, 1920
Introduction and popularization of specialized instruments	C. Kielland, 1915 (midpelvic rotation)
	L. G. Barton, 1925 (transverse arrest)
	E. B. Piper, 1929 (aftercoming head)
Refinement and popularization of vacuum extraction	T. Malmström, 1956

of obstetrics can still profit from reviewing the original papers and descriptions of these innovators. Despite the introduction of electronic and biochemical monitoring, the process of parturition still involves powers, passages, and a passenger—and in carefully selected cases some form of assistance in delivery will always be required.

REFERENCES

1. Dumont M. Histoire et petite historie du forceps. J Gynecol Obstet Biol Reprod (Paris) 1984; 13:743–757.
2. Spink MS, Lewis GL. Albucasis on surgery and instruments. Berkeley, CA: University of California Press, 1973: 494.
3. Guthrie D. A history of medicine. London: Thomas Nelson & Sons, Ltd, 1945.
4. Mauriceau F. Traité des maladies de femmes grosses. Quatrième Edition, Paris: D'Houry, L., 1694.
5. Das K. Obstetric forceps: its history and evolution. Calcutta: The Art Press, 1929.
6. Aveling JA. The Chamberlens and the midwifery forceps. Memorials of the family and an essay on the invention of the instrument. London: Churchill, 1882.
7. Speert H. The obstetric forceps. Clin Obstet Gynecol 1960; 3:761–766.
8. Drinkwater H. The modern descendants of Dr. Peter Chamberlen. The Liverpool Medico-Chirurg J 1916; 69:98-105.
9. Gordon BL. Medieval and renaissance medicine. New York: Philosophical Library, 1959.
10. Ingraham CB. The Chamberlens and the obstetrical forceps. Am J. Obstet Dis Women Child 1911; 63:827–849.
11. Mettler CC, Mettler FA. History of medicine. Philadelphia: The Blakiston Co., 1947.
12. Drinkwater KR. The midwifery forceps: historical sketch. Liverpool

Medico-Chirurg J 1913; 64:451–465.
13. Martius G. Operative obstetrics. 12th ed. New York: Thieme-Stratton, 1980.
14. Dill LV. The obstetrical forceps. Springfield, IL: Charles C Thomas, 1953.
15. Rhodes P. Edmund Chapman (fl. 1735). J Obstet Gynaecol Br Commonw 1968; 75:793–799.
16. Ramsbotham FH, Keating WV. The principles and practice of obstetric medicine and surgery in reference to the process of parturition. Philadelphia: Blanchard & Lea, 1861.
17. Benion E. Antique medical instruments. Berkeley, CA: University of California Press, 1979: 127.
18. Douglass RG, Stromme WB. Operative obstetrics. 3rd ed. New York: Appleton-Century-Crofts, 1976.
19. Thierry E. Les spatules: manoeuvre du toboggan (LeT.). Presse Med 1960; 68:317–319.
20. Laufe LE. Obstetric forceps. New York: Harper & Row, 1968.
21. Major RH. A history of medicine. 2nd ed. Springfield, IL: Charles C Thomas, 1954.
22. Smellie W. Anatomical tables of the practice of midwifery. London, 1754.
23. Andrews HR. William Hunter and his work in midwifery. Br Med J 1915; 1:277–281.
24. Lasky II. John Hunter, the Shakespeare of medicine. Surg Gynecol Obstet 1983; 156:511–518.
25. Richardson OR, Evans MI, Cibils LA. Midforceps delivery: a critical review. Am J Obstet Gynecol 1983; 145:621–632.
26. Dewhurst J. Royal confinements: a gynaecological history of Britain's royal family. New York: St. Martin's Press, 1980: 115.
27. Holland E. The Princess Charlotte of Wales: a triple obstetric tragedy. J Obstet Gynaecol Br Emp 1951; 58:905–919.
28. Pearse WH. "And, having writ, moves on." Am J Obstet Gynecol 1983; 146:233–236.
29. Huard P. Sciences, Médecine, pharmacie de la revolution à l'Empire (1789–1815). Paris: Roger Dacosta, 1970: 223.
30. Edmonson JM, Truax, C. Mechanics of surgery [Reprint]. San Francisco: Norman Publishing, 1987.
31. Davis AD. The development of anesthesia. Am Sci 1982; 70:522–528.
32. Leavitt JW. "Science" enters the birthing room: obstetrics in America since the eighteenth century. J Am Hist 1983; 70:281–303.
33. Witkowski GJ. Histoire des accouchements chez tous les peuples. Havre: Lamale et Cie, 1877.
34. Burrell HL, Tucker GR. Aseptic surgery. Boston Med Surg 1889; 121:329–334.
35. Coues WP. Sir James W. Simpson (1811–1870) the prince of obstetricians. N Engl. J Med 1928; 199:221–224.
36. Jones OP. A bench mark for obstetric history in the United States. Obstet Gynecol 1974; 43:784–791.
37. Roberts RB. General analgesia and anesthesia. In: Abouleish, E., ed. Pain control in obstetrics. Philadelphia: JB Lippincott, 1977: 367.
38. Francis SW. Biographical sketch of Professor George T. Elliott (sic) M.D. Med Surg Rep 1871; 24:179–180.
39. Forster FMC. Robert Barnes and his obstetric forceps. Aust NZ J Obstet Gynaecol 1971; 11:139–147.
40. Longo LD, Hodge HL. Dictionary of American medical biography. Westport, CT: Greenwood Press, 1984.
41. Pajot C. Travaux d'obstétrique et de gynécologie, précédés d'éléments de practique obstétricale, Paris, H. Lauwereynes, 1882.
42. Obituary, Professor Pajot. Br Med J 1896; 2:538.
43. Necrologie, M. Le Pr Pajot (de Paris). Le Progres Med 1896; 2:78.
44. Discours prononcé aux obseques du Professor Pajot au nom de la Faculté de Médecine. Ann Gynecol 1896; 45:1.
45. Luikart R. A modification of the Kielland, Simpson, and Tucker-McLane forceps to simplify their use and improve function in safety. Am J Obstet Gynecol 1937; 34:686-687.
46. Scanzoni, FW. Lehrbuch der geburtshilfe. 3rd ed. Vienna: Seidel, 1885.
47. Dennon EH. Forcep deliveries. 2nd ed. Philadelphia: FA Davis, 1964.
48. Bill AH. A new axis traction handle

for solid blade forceps. Am J Obstet Gynecol 1925; 9:606–607.

49. Parry-Jones EJ. Barton's forceps. Baltimore: Williams & Wilkins, 1972.
50. Barton LG, Caldwell WE, Studdiford WE. A new obstetric forceps. Am J Obstet Gynecol 1928; 15:16–26.
51. Kielland C. Uber die anlegung der zange am nicht rotierten kopf mit beschreibung eines neuen zangenmodelles und einer neuen anlegungsmethode. Monatssch Geburtsh Gynakol 1916; 43:38–78.
52. Speert, H. Obstetrics and gynecology in America. A history. Baltimore: Waverly Press, Inc, 1980.
53. DeLee JB. The prophylactic forceps operation. Am J Obstet Gynecol 1920; 1:34–44.
54. Piper EB, Bachman C. The prevention of fetal injuries in breech delivery. JAMA 1929; 92:217–221.
55. Chalmers JA. James Young Simpson and the "suction-tractor." J Obstet Gynaecol Br Commonw 1963; 70:94–100.
56. Chalmers JA. The ventouse: the obstetric vacuum extractor. Chicago: Year Book, 1971.
57. Sjöstedt JE. The vacuum extractor and forceps in obstetrics: a clinical study. Acta Obstet Gynecol Scand 1967; 46(suppl 10):3–208.
58. Malmström T. The vacuum extractor. An obstetrical instrument and the parturiometer, a tokographic device. Acta Obstet Gynecol Scand 1957; 36(suppl 3):7–87.
59. Malmström T. Jansson I. Use of the vacuum extractor. Clin Obstet Gynecol 1965; 8:893–913.
60. Thiery M. Obstetric vacuum extraction. Obstet Gynecol Annu 1985; 14:73–111.
61. Hildanus. Guilhelmi fabricii Hildani opera. Frankfurt-on-Main, 1632.
62. Johnson T. The workes of that famous chirurgion A. Parey. London, 1665: 243.
63. Younge J. An account of balls of hair taken from the uterus and ovaria of several women. Philos Trans R Soc Lond 1706–1707; 25:2387.
64. Duns J. A memoir of Sir James Y. Simpson. Edinborough, 1873: 288.
65. Guidicelli. Rev Med Franc 1847; I:126.
66. Arnott N. Elements of physics or natural philosophy, general and medical, explained independently of technical mathematics and containing new disquisitions and practical suggestions. London, Longman Rees, 1827.
67. Malmström T. Vacuum extractor. An obstetrical instrument. Acta Obstet Gynaecol Scand 1954; 33(suppl 4):3.
68. Willett JA. The treatment of placenta praevia by continuous weight traction—a report of seven cases. Proc R Soc Med 1925; 18:90–94.
69. Lovset J. Modern techniques of vaginal operative delivery in cephalic presentation. Acta Obstet Gynecol Scand 1965; 44:102–106.
70. Party M. Ventouses obstetricales. La V.O.F., Ventouse Obstetricale Française. Paris: Vigot Freres, 1966.
71. Saling E, Rothe J. Modifikation der vakuumextraktionsvorrichtung. Z. Geburtshilfe Perinatol 1978; 182:93–95.
72. O'Neil AGB, Skull E, Michael C. A new method of traction for the vacuum cup. Aust NZ J Obstet Gynecol 1981; 21:24–25.
73. Bird GC. The new generation in vacuum extractor—Bird manual. Gothenburg, Sweden: AB Vacuum Extractor, 1983.
74. Halkin V. Une modification de la ventouse de Malmström. Bull Soc R Belge Gynecol d'Obstet 1964; 34:145–150.
75. Bird GC. Modification of Malmström's vacuum extractor. Br Med J 1969; 3:526.
76. Pelosi MA, Apuzzio J. Use of the soft, silicone obstetric vacuum cup for the delivery of the fetal head at cesarean section. J Reprod Med 1984; 29:289–292.
77. Wood JF. An evaluation of a new plastic disposable vacuum extractor cup. J Am Osteopath Assoc 1969; 66:1251–1254.
78. Paul RH, Staisch KJ, Pine SN. The "new" vacuum extractor. Obstet Gynecol 1973; 41:800–802.
79. Laufe LE. A new divergent outlet forceps. Am J Obstet Gynecol 1968; 101:509–512.

2

Instruments and Indications

*There are many who believe that the delivery of women is easy
... and in truth there is no mystery when things go normally. But,
when an accouchement is preternatural it becomes the most
difficult, laborious and dangerous of all surgical procedures.*
FRANÇOIS MAURICEAU, 1694 (1)

*... Branche gauche à la main gauche,
à gauche la première;
tout doit être gauche,
sauf l'accoucheur ...*
CHARLES PAJOT, 1882 (2)

Introduction: The Obstetric Armamentarium

Modern obstetric forceps consist of a set of forged steel blades
with a cephalic curve and usually a pelvic curve. The blades commonly articulate or cross in a lock except in certain specialized instruments. Each pair is a unique set and each is numbered; thus, blades are
not interchangeable. Various forceps differ in construction of one or
more of the components of blade, shank, lock, or handle. Each model
was designed in response to a specific set of clinical management
problems and/or for convenience of the operator.

Forceps consist of three major parts: handles, lock, and blades
(Figs. 2.1 and 2.2). The handles on modern instruments are hollowed
to conserve weight and may incorporate finger guides or rests in their
construction, adjacent to the lock. Some instruments, such as Kielland
forceps, still retain a vestige of curvature in the tips of the handles, a
remnant of the obstetric hook or crochet (see Fig. 1.9). In the heroic era
of vaginal delivery, cesarean section was uncommon and dangerous. If
accouchement with forceps was unsuccessful or the fetal lie prevented
their application, the instrument could be reversed and the hook incor-

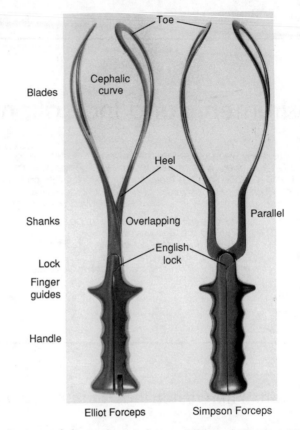

Elliot Forceps   Simpson Forceps

Figure 2.1.   Anatomy of classic obstetric forceps (Elliot and Simpson) (1).

porated in the handle brought into use. Some 19th century forceps handles had removable covers on such hooks to avoid maternal or operator trauma while the crochet was not required. In other models the hooked ends of the handles were retained but they were nonfunctional except as traction assists (see Fig. 1.9). In modern instruments, the curved tips of the handles were brought upward adjacent to the

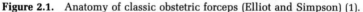

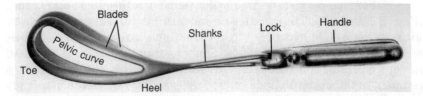

Figure 2.2.   Anatomy of classic obstetric forceps. Lateral view of Simpson forceps (1). Note pelvic curve of the fenestrated blades.

lock and made into the finger rests. The late 19th century French accoucheur, C. Pajot, is said to have pointed out the curved ends of the forceps during his lectures, telling his students that the hooks had been left on the handles as a reminder to obstetricians never to use them!

Standard forceps overlap or articulate in the lock (3). A number of standard lock systems exist, reflecting in part the long history of forceps development. Lock mechanisms have both practical and simply conservative reasons for continued use. The most common articulation for classical outlet forceps such as the Elliot and Simpson models is the *English lock*. This lock was invented from earlier models by William Smellie in the early 19th century (Fig. 2.3). This mechanism is a simple and ingenious invention consisting of dual machined

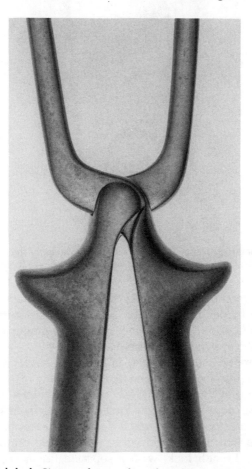

Figure 2.3. English lock. Simpson forceps (here depicted partially disarticulated).

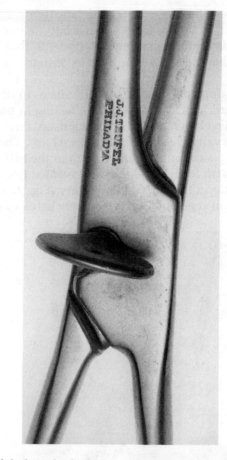

Figure 2.4.   French lock. Hodge forceps (ca. 1833). (Courtesy of the Dittrick Museum of Medical History, Historical Division/Cleveland Health Sciences Library, Cleveland, OH.)

grooves in the forceps shanks. This lock provides a secure articulation yet leaves the blades immediately free for repositioning when separated by lateral motion. The design's survival to modern times and use in dozens of forceps models attests to its utility.

The *French lock* (Fig. 2.4) is the simplest, consisting of two flattened shank surfaces approximated by a screw or pin. Few instruments in use in the United States incorporate this locking mechanism. The illustration depicts a Hodge forceps, dating from the early 19th century based on the classic French design of Levret (4).

The *German lock* combines an articulation pin or screw, similar to that of a French lock, with a separate finger screw that abuts against a slotted metal post, firmly securing the blades together (Fig.

2.5). Except for axis traction instruments, such as DeWees or Tarnier forceps, this lock is uncommonly encountered. The German lock produces the most secure articulation of any locking mechanism but this great strength is accompanied by inflexibility and an increase in compression force against the fetal head.

The *sliding lock* (Fig. 2.6) is a relatively recent innovation by Boerma in 1907 (4) subsequently popularized by Kielland (5). The ability to alter the point of blade articulation is important in instruments designed for midpelvic procedures where cranial asynclitism is common. Forceps designed for use in midpelvic rotation, such as the Kielland and Barton forceps, incorporate this lock design.

Other uncommonly encountered instruments use special lock or articulation systems (see Martius (6)).

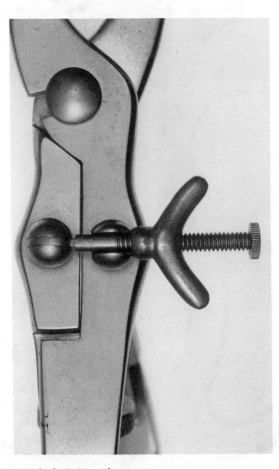

Figure 2.5.   German lock. DeWees forceps.

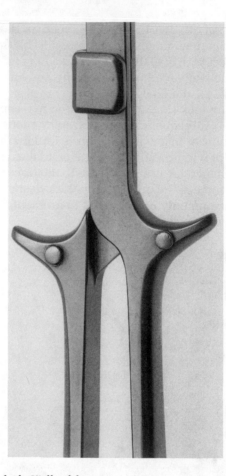

Figure 2.6.   Sliding lock. Kielland forceps.

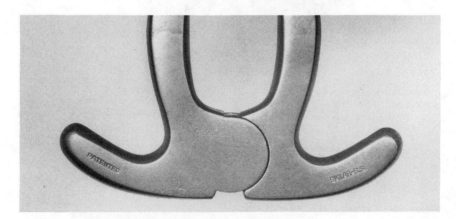

Figure 2.7.   Pivot lock. Laufe forceps.

The *pivot lock* is the most unusual and was designed for use with the divergent blade forceps of Laufe (Fig. 2.7). A two-bladed cavity machined into the handle of the forceps incorporates a central pin upon which the slotted protrusion of the second blade articulates. In this unique forceps design, the shanks of the blades do not overlap and the only contact between the left and right parts of the instrument is via the lock mechanism itself.

The parallel shanks of Shute forceps are joined not by a specific lock mechanism but by means of a threaded bolt held in place on one shaft of the forceps by a wing nut. The Naegele forceps uses a composite locking mechanism combining features of the French and English models. Finally, the Baumberger divergent forceps articulates the shanks with a peg on the left forceps shank fitted into a hole on the right shank. These and other unique designs were invented to reduce compression of the fetal head (6).

Classic Forceps: Simpson and Elliot

The most successful obstetric forceps are the designs originally developed by James Young Simpson (1842) (Fig. 2.8) and George L. Elliot, Jr. (1858) (Fig. 2.9). Both are highly versatile instruments that can be applied in many clinical settings. These forceps are most commonly used for elective outlet applications or lower pelvic rotations. But, in skilled hands these classic blades perform virtually any of the required instrumental deliveries and can be used interchangeably. The survival of both designs is a tribute to medical conservatism and the success of the initial design.

Both instruments incorporate cephalic and pelvic curves but differ in several respects. The shanks of the Simpson forceps diverge abruptly as they leave the handles. The space theoretically allows insertion of the operator's middle finger, providing a cushion to mini-

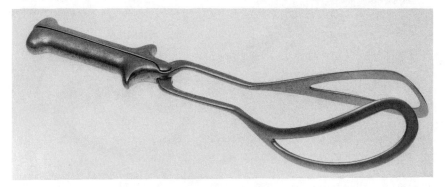

Figure 2.8. Simpson forceps (ca. 1842).

mize and control the compression of the fetal head. Such control is, however, at best difficult to regulate. Both the Simpson and Elliot forceps are classified by length of the blades as long (18 inches or longer) or short (15 inches). The Elliot long forceps is slightly longer than the Simpson long, and there is somewhat less distance between the blade tips (3, 7).

The major differences between the instruments concern the shape of the cephalic curve, the position of the shanks, and the construction of the handle. Simpson forceps have a more elongated and flattened cephalic curve combined with the nonoverlapping or parallel shanks. When Simpson forceps are fully articulated, there is no truly effective means of controlling cranial compression unless a towel or sponge is placed between the handles to separate them—a technique routinely practiced by some accoucheurs. The elongated cephalic curve and the wide shanks make Simpson forceps best suited for well-molded heads of term-size infants. The widely separated shanks of the Simpson forceps are least traumatic in traction through a multiparous introitus but are less desirable for major rotations or in use in women with a narrow introitus than Elliot-design instruments because of separation of the shanks.

Elliot forceps have overlapping shanks and a more rounded cephalic curve. The instrument includes a finger-activated screw mechanism in the handle to help limit the extent of cranial compression when the blades are articulated and traction is applied, eliminating the need for a folded towel. The modifications to the blades and shank make Elliot's instrument better suited than Simpson's for rotational deliveries. With rotation, especially when applied to nulliparous patients, the narrower, overlapping shanks of the Elliot instru-

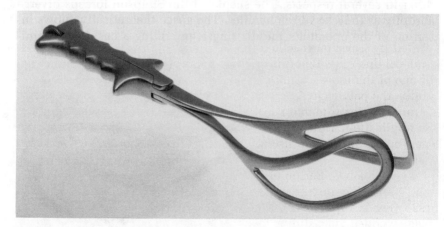

Figure 2.9. Elliot forceps (ca. 1858).

ment are less likely to injure the introitus. In theory at least, the smaller, more rounded cephalic curve of the blades of the Elliot forceps is less ideal than Simpson's design for application to heavily molded fetal heads because the ends of the blades produce pressure points on the fetal scalp at the narrower distance between the tips of the blades.

Modified Classic Instruments

The most popular of the modified classic instruments is the Tucker-McLane forceps (Fig. 2.10), which is an Elliot-type forceps design with extended shanks and solid, nonfenestrated blades. The blades are frequently manufactured with pseudofenestration, an ingenious modification first suggested in 1850 by A. Hohl and reintroduced and popularized by Luikart (8–10). In pseudofenestration, the central portion of the blade is thinned or hollowed providing an indentation that permits the blade to more firmly grasp the fetal head in a fashion similar to an actual fenestrated blade. At the same time, however, the ease of insertion and rotation characteristic of solid-bladed instruments is retained (Fig. 2.11). Solid blades are in general easier to insert and less likely to result in marks on the fetal head. In contrast, solid blades, unless pseudofenestrated, are also more likely to slip during traction than fenestrated blades, with enhanced risk of maternal/fetal laceration. The design of the Tucker-McLane makes them most useful as midpelvic rotators.

Specialized Instruments

In this category are a variety of instruments with design modifications for use in special clinical circumstances.

The most familiar specialized forceps is the instrument invented by Christian Kielland in 1915 (Fig. 2.12) (5). This forceps is unusual due to two modifications. First, a sliding lock is used instead of one of the more common methods of affixing the shanks, and secondly, the pelvic curve is essentially absent. The second modification permits the instrument to be used as a midpelvic rotator and facilitates its application. However, these modifications also make the instrument more difficult to use safely, especially for the less experienced operator.

Lyman G. Barton of Plattsburgh, New York presented his unusual appearing instrument to the American Gynecological Club in 1925 (Fig. 2.13) (11, 12). These forceps consist of a hinged anterior blade wedged via a sliding lock to a sharply angulated posterior blade. Their unusual appearance is due to their original design intention to

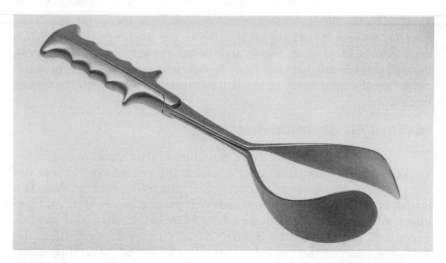

Figure 2.10.   Tucker-McLane forceps.

assist delivery in high transverse arrests. Barton forceps are uncommonly applied, but are by no means difficult to use once the operator has mastered the wandering application of the anterior blade and techniques of insertion for the posterior one. However, great care must be taken during rotations with Barton forceps, as the length of the shanks/handles and the angle of articulation between the plane of the blades and handle permit great force to be generated if rotation is vigorous. A

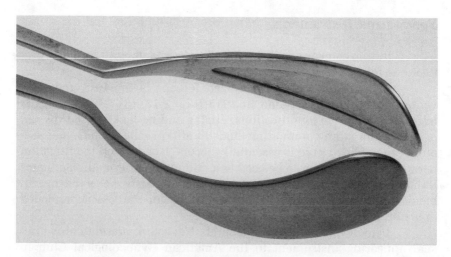

Figure 2.11.   Pseudofenestration of the forceps blade. Note the hollowed central portion of the blade (Luikart modification) (5, 6).

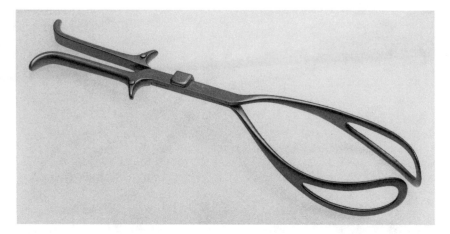

Figure 2.12.   Kielland forceps (ca. 1916). Note sliding lock and absence of a pelvic curve.

modified Kielland-Barton forceps has also been described, combining blades of changeable angle. Locked in the appropriate position, the forceps can function as either instrument (13).

Piper forceps have only a single application—the aftercoming head in a breech delivery (Fig. 2.14) (14). This instrument consists of a long forceps with flexible shanks, fenestrated blades, and an English lock. The forceps is specifically designed to stabilize and protect the fetal head during breech delivery.

Other specialized divergent or parallel instruments have been described by Laufe (Fig. 2.15) (15), Shute, and many others. Both the Laufe and Shute (16) instruments were designed to reduce fetal cranial

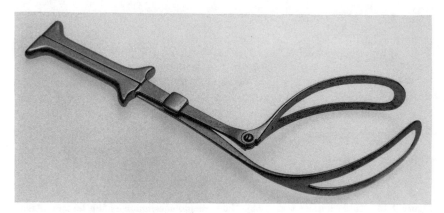

Figure 2.13.   Barton forceps (ca. 1925).

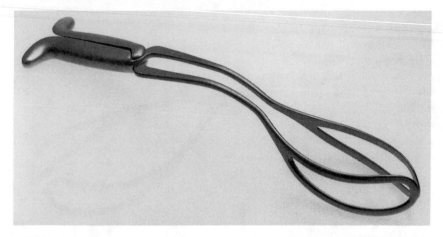

Figure 2.14. Piper forceps (ca. 1929). Note long shanks and their special curvature facilitating application in breech deliveries.

compression. Both designs are primarily useful as outlet forceps, although rotations can be performed with Laufe's parallel blade instrument (17). Many other forceps designs exist, the majority being modifications of these standard designs (6).

Axis Traction

Forceps incorporating axis traction date to the late 19th century when Tarnier and Pajot emphasized the techniques of traction in the pelvic curve (Carus' curve) as important in successful instrumental

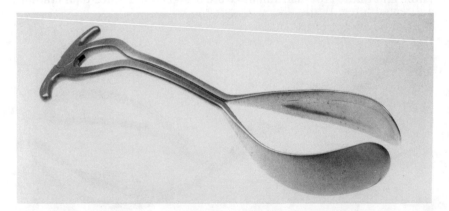

Figure 2.15. Laufe forceps (ca. 1968). Note pseudofenestration of the forceps blade (Luikart modification) and the pivot lock mechanism.

delivery. Although axis traction instruments are not currently popular, most services still retain one or more of the various models. The De-Wees instrument is an example of this type (Fig. 2.16). In this forceps, a Simpson-type forceps is fitted with a German lock and an arching, modified shank that leads to a handle combined with a universal joint. Such instruments are derivations of the Tarnier design and in general are inflexible devices that are somewhat clumsy for most clinicians to apply—a problem no doubt complicated by the fact that such instruments are rarely used and many modern accoucheurs are inexperienced with their assembly and correct application (7).

The Hawk-Dennen instrument is an unusually clever modification of a standard outlet type forceps in which the axis traction principle is incorporated into the design by the simple expedient of changing the angle between the plane of the shanks and blade (7).

Recognizing the desirability of axis traction, but the limitations of the Tarnier design, Bill designed a traction handle to be applied to any standard outlet forceps (18). A curved metal case designed to fit over the finger guard and shanks of a Simpson- or Elliot-type forceps was connected to a rod, articulating with a traction handle. A small metal pointer was positioned at the articulation of the handle and rod, serving to indicate the correct angle for traction (Fig. 2.17). If axis traction is desired, Bill's handle is a most convenient device to use, as it is applicable to standard forceps and does not rigidly lock or approximate the handles as do the various Tarnier-type instruments.

Modern disinterest in axis traction instruments stems from their original design intention, i.e., more effective traction. When Tarnier developed his design, overcoming relative cephalopelvic disproportion was desirable. His design permitted the most efficient use of directed force. While the emphasis on axis traction is still perfectly valid, the concept of instrumental assistance overcoming dystocia by

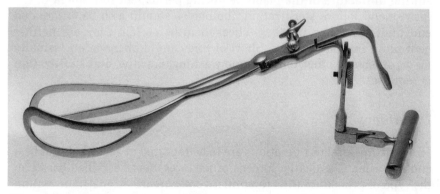

Figure 2.16. DeWees axis traction forceps.

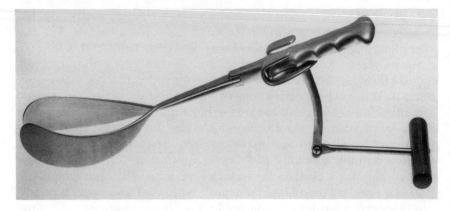

Figure 2.17.   Axis traction handle of Bill applied to Tucker-McLane forceps. Note *indication arrow* and the *inscribed line* on the traction bar indicating the correct angle for traction.

externally applied force is not. Further, the German lock of the De-Wees and other such instruments excessively compresses the fetal head. There is little current use for these instruments.

For interested readers an extensive discussion of the physics of forceps application with emphasis on forces generated during delivery are found in Laufe's text (3).

Most modern forceps are constructed of highly polished stainless steel and when properly cared for will last nearly indefinitely. Like any surgical instrument, forceps deserve careful attention during sterilization and wrapping. Following use and before repacking for sterilization, each pair should be carefully examined, with special attention to the blades. Either through repeated heat sterilizations or episodes of dropping, cracks can develop in the metal, eventually resulting in fracture of the blade, requiring permanent retirement of the instrument. Before sterilization, the blades should also be articulated and their enscribed numbers checked to be certain they are neither bent nor a mismatched set. Short of this careful observation virtually no maintenance other than routine washing, packing, and sterilization is required.

Definitions

How forceps operations are to be reported or recorded is at best controversial. Classically, forceps procedures were described based on the type of procedure (i.e., rotational versus nonrotational), the station of the fetal head (high, mid, outlet) and the urgency of the indication (elective versus indicated). In the attempt to better describe the difficulty of applications, a coding system was developed in the early 1950s reporting the type of procedure, dependent upon the station of the fetal head (19). Most practicing American obstetricians were taught to code the station of forceps procedures as high, high mid, low mid, or low (outlet) operations. Each of these positions reflected a stage in the expected mechanism of labor and corresponded to a specific or convenient anatomic pelvic plane.

In the attempt to standardize reporting and practice, the American College of Obstetricians and Gynecologists (ACOG) periodically reviews obstetric forceps procedures and issues guidelines. The most recent statement (1988) represents a departure from the prior definitions (1972) and identifies three types of forceps operations: *midforceps, low forceps,* and *outlet forceps* (Tables 2.1–2.5) (20).

Outlet forceps operations are now defined as the application of forceps under conditions of full cervical dilation, the fetal head having reached the pelvic floor, with the scalp visible at the introitus without separating the labia and with the saggital suture in the anteroposterior diameter of the pelvic outlet or at an obliquity not exceeding 45° from the vertical. Other applications, when the fetal head is engaged but the conditions for outlet forceps are not met, are considered as either low forceps or midforceps operations.

These new definitions distinguish between two types of low forceps operations, specifically those with minimal (<45°) or substantial (>45°) rotation. Remaining procedures with or without rotation at stations above +2 are coded as midforceps operations, with specific qualification (Tables 2.2 and 2.3).

These definitions are an improvement on the prior 1972 guidelines in which no distinction in coding was made between *anatomically* midpelvic extractions (previously the high mid and mid) and the much easier and less risky lower pelvic rotational or nonrotational deliveries. Under the 1972 definition, *any* rotation at any level constituted a midforceps procedure. The 1972 rules were instituted at a time when serious concern was raised about the appropriateness of *any* midpelvic procedure, without distinction of difficulty or corresponding maternal-fetal risk.

Station

One of the most taxing of clinical evaluations is the accurate determination of station of the fetal head. Station is commonly reported as the lowest level reached by the bony presenting part of the fetal head, measured against the imaginary midpelvic plane of least

Table 2.1.   ACOG Definitions: Forceps Operations, 1988[a]

Outlet forceps—the application of forceps when:
  The scalp is visible at the introitus without spreading the labia
  The fetal skull has reached the pelvic floor
  The sagittal suture is in the anterior/posterior diameter or in the right or left occiput
    anterior or posterior position
  The fetal head is at or on the perineum
Low forceps—the application of forceps when the leading point of the skull is at station
  +2 or more. There are two subdivisions:[b]
  Rotation is 45° or less
  Rotation is more than 45°
Midforceps—the application of forceps when the fetal head is engaged but the leading
  point of the skull is above station +2

[a]From Committee on Obstetrics: Maternal and Fetal Medicine 59: Obstetric Forceps. American College of Obstetricians and Gynecologists, Washington, DC: 1988.
[b]Station is defined as the distance *in centimeters* between the leading bony portion of the fetal skull and the plane of the maternal ischial spines.

dimensions, which passes between the ischial spines. The distance toward or away from the perineum is measured in centimeters or in thirds. Stations below the plane of the spines are described as "plus" or positive, those above as "minus" or negative.

The new ACOG definitions require that station now be reported in *centimeters*, a departure from prior practice for most practitioners and a move that may prove more troublesome than helpful, at least initially.

When the cranium of a term fetus enters the maternal pelvis and the biparietal diameter passes through the pelvic brim, *engagement* is said to have occurred, that is, the fetal head is fixed in the pelvic inlet. Clinically, engagement is verified during maternal abdominal palpation by noting that the operator's hands cannot easily displace the fetal head from the pelvis during Leopold's maneuvers. Engagement can also be evaluated by pelvic examination or by real time ultrasound and, classically, by x-ray pelvimetry. In the anatomically normal pelvis, the fetal head enters as an occiput transverse, with the left occiput transverse (LOT) position predominating. In the *unmolded* fetal head, the mean distance from the leading edge of the scalp to the midplane of the fetal head (biparietal diameter) is approximately 5 cm. As this distance is half the usual depth of the maternal pelvis, with

Table 2.2.   ACOG Definitions: Qualifications of Midforceps Operations, 1988[a]

Under very unusual circumstances, such as the sudden onset of severe fetal or maternal compromise, application of forceps above station +2 may be attempted while simultaneously initiating preparations for a cesarean delivery in the event the forceps maneuver is unsuccessful. Under no circumstances, however, should forceps be applied to an unengaged presenting part or when the cervix is not completely dilated.[b]

[a]From Committee on Obstetrics: Maternal and Fetal Medicine 59: Obstetric Forceps. American College of Obstetricians and Gynecologists, Washington, DC: 1988.
[b]Station is defined as the distance *in centimeters* between the leading bony portion of the fetal skull and the plane of the maternal ischial spines.

Table 2.3. ACOG Definitions: Conditions Required for Midforceps Operations, 1988[a]

An experienced person performing or supervising the procedure
An assessment of maternal-fetal size relationship
Adequate anesthesia
Willingness to abandon the attempt if the forceps procedure does not proceed easily

[a]From Committee on Obstetrics: Maternal and Fetal Medicine 59: Obstetric Forceps. American College of Obstetricians and Gynecologists, Washington, DC: 1988.

engagement the bony presenting part of the head reaches the level of the ischial spines, defined as zero station. Applications to the fetal head above this level are *high forceps* and are not justified. Attempts at accouchement from stations below engagement but less than +2 are uncommonly justified except in trials of forceps or vacuum by the most experienced of practitioners (Table 2.3).

The determination of station is subjective, and considerable variation between observers occurs. This fact alone makes the use of centimeters from the spines for the diagnosis of station questionable. The diagnosis of station also varies if examinations are conducted with or without uterine contractions. Confounding problems are filling or nonfilling of the hollow of the sacrum by the fetal head and confusion brought about by asynclitism, caput formation, and cranial molding (7). The fetal head is often a relatively tight fit to the maternal pelvis. The process of labor with its recurrent contractions, augmented by maternal voluntary efforts, remolds the fetal head into the classic elongate shape, fitting the architecture of the birth canal but also distorting cranial landmarks. These issues are of great clinical importance as progress in labor is judged by cervical dilatation and descent of the fetal head with accompanying rotation. The real issue in palpating for station is the locale of the largest diameter of the fetal head—the biparietal diameter.

In the consideration of revising the existing ACOG coding recommendations for indications for forceps operations, several important points were raised. The reviewers recognized that protracted labor potentially places a fetus at increased risk. However, previous recommendations about the acceptable length of the second stage are no longer valid. In the era before electronic monitoring, clinical studies indicated a higher fetal risk for morbidity and mortality when the second stage of labor exceeded an arbitrary limit, usually defined as 2 hours. However, with modern electronic monitoring and other means of fetal surveillance, rigid application of the 2-hour rule is no longer defensible (21). As is discussed elsewhere in the text, the common use of epidural anesthesia has been partially responsible for altering clinical decisions concerning the appropriate length of the second stage of labor. Thus, modern definitions for a prolonged second stage are only approximate and should *not* be considered as rigid indica-

Table 2.4.   ACOG Definitions: Recording of Forceps Operations, 1988[a]

The indications for the forceps operation, including the position and station of the vertex at the time of application of the forceps, should be specified in a detailed operative description in the patient's medical record.[b]

[a]From Committee on Obstetrics: Maternal and Fetal Medicine 59: Obstetric Forceps. American College of Obstetricians and Gynecologists, Washington, DC: 1988.
[b]Station is defined as the distance *in centimeters* between the leading bony portion of the fetal skull and the plane of the maternal ischial spines.

tions for intervention. These limits for a primigravida are more than 3 hours in the second stage, if a regional anesthetic has been given, or more than 2 hours in the absence of regional anesthesia. The time limits for the multipara are more than 2 hours in the second stage, if regional anesthesia has been administered, and more than 1 hour if it has not (Table 2.5). *When these limits are exceeded, this is not an immediate indication for operative intervention but a time at which the risks and benefits of allowing labor to continue spontaneously or to be assisted are assessed and documented.* Uncommonly with fetal and maternal compromise, applications of forceps above +2 station may be required. In general, it is recommended that these applications be attempted only while preparations for cesarean section are simultaneously initiated (Table 2.2). *Forceps should never be applied to an unengaged presenting part (high forceps) or when the cervix is not completely dilated.*

Documentation

Although not specifically stated in the 1988 ACOG definitions, given the medical/legal climate in which we practice and the variations in routine recording of forceps use, in the author's opinion, *all operative or instrumental deliveries should be dictated in the same fashion as any surgical procedure* (Table 2.4). The dictation includes a statement of the indications for the procedure, the anesthesia used, personnel involved, and an outline of the actual procedure. A careful

Table 2.5.   ACOG Definitions: Indications for Forceps Operations, 1988[a]

Shortening the second stage of labor[b]
Prolonged second stage of labor
  Primigravidas—more than 3 hours with a regional anesthetic or more than 2 hours
    without a regional anesthetic
  Multiparas—more than 2 hours with a regional anesthesia or more than 1 hour without
    a regional anesthetic[c]
Fetal distress
Maternal indications[c]

[a]From Committee on Obstetrics: Maternal and Fetal Medicine 59: Obstetric Forceps. American College of Obstetricians and Gynecologists, Washington, DC: 1988.
[b]As long as the criteria for outlet forceps are met (see Table 2.1).
[c]Exhaustion, cardiac problems, etc.

discussion of the reasons for the application with a rapid review of the clinical circumstances is appropriate. The type of instruments, difficulties in insertion, and the station, position, and deflection of the fetal head should all be recorded. A statement should be made as to necessity for rotation, if performed, and the difficulty of the extraction. Additional complications including shoulder dystocia, episiotomy extension or maternal-fetal lacerations and their repair and an estimate of blood loss should be included. These requirements assist in statistical analysis of forceps applications and ultimately serve to protect both the institution and the accoucheur.

Indications for Forceps Use

Introduction

The indications for the application of forceps vary, with important differences in practice between institutions and among practitioners. Not surprisingly, the disparity between European and American obstetric practice is reflected in major differences in the indications for and incidence of forceps application and vacuum extraction (see Tables 2.5 and 2.6). In 1920, DeLee suggested "prophylactic" application of forceps in the second stage of labor as a means of reducing both maternal trauma and fetal risk and strongly influenced thereafter the use of instrumental delivery in American obstetrics (38). Many, if not most, American obstetricians were trained to view instrumental delivery as the norm of obstetrical conduct. The concept of prophylactic forceps still lives on today in the common use of instrumental delivery in patients who receive epidural anesthesia or experience delayed descent when the second stage of labor is extended beyond the 2-hour limit enshrined in traditional obstetric teaching (see Table 2.5).

Fetal Distress

The immediate need for delivery is a classic indication for forceps use (Tables 2.5 and 2.7). Occult cord prolapse, abruptio placentae, cord entanglements, and similar obstetric disasters result in fetal bradycardia and the requirement for prompt delivery. There is no question that in these and similar circumstances prompt accouchement is necessary to avoid serious or fatal fetal injury. Classically, fetal distress was established by observation of meconium passage and/or

Table 2.6. Statistics on Forceps Use

Reference	Type of Forceps	Years of Study (Country)	Total Deliveries	Forceps Deliveries	Incidence Forceps (%)	Comparison Figures (%)
Bergman & Malmström (22)	All	1958–1960 (Sweden)	90,005	990	1.1	VE = 1.8[a] CS = 1.8
Cooke (23)	All	1960–1965 (Canada)	7,019	2,288	32.6	CS = 7.2
Widen et al. (24)	All	1961–1964 (U.S.)	20,056	5,545	27.6	CS = 7.8 VE = 1.0
Leeton & Waldron (25)	All	1969 (U.S.)	4,832	720	14.9	
Cardozo et al. (26)	All	1980–1981 (U.S.)	2,708	336	12.4	CS = 7.2
Decker et al. (27)	Mid	1940–1951 (U.S.)	21,857	547	2.5	
Cosgrove et al. (28)	Mid	NR (U.S.)	52,631	1,000	1.9	CS = 3.6
Kirk et al. (29)	Mid	1956–1957 (U.S.)	6,043	254	4.2	CS = 2.8
Danforth & Ellis (30)	Mid	1955–1961	14,780	1,907		
Nyirjesy et al. (31)	Low	1961 (U.S.)	29,186	11,674	40	
Cooke (23)	Mid	1960–1965 (U.S.)	7,019	426	6.8	CS = 9.3
Dunlop (32)	Mid	1965–1967 (Canada)	5,633	292	5.2	
Bowes & Bowes (33)	Mid		6,331	71	1.2	
Dierker et al. (34)	Mid	1976–1982	21,414	176	0.8	CS = 9.3
Nilsen (35)	All	1981	NR	NR	3.8	VE = 3.2
Bergsjo et al. (36)	All	1979 (Czecho-slovakia	NR	NR	1.3	CS = 4.0
		1979 (Denmark)	NR	NR	0.7	CS = 10.3
		1979 (Finland)	NR	NR	0.3	CS = 11.9
		1976 (France)	NR	NR	8.0	CS = 8.0
		NR (Hungary)	NR	NR	0.4	CS = 8.0
		1978 (Nether-lands)	NR	NR	1.7	CS = 3.6
		1979 (Norway)	NR	NR	3.2	CS = 8.0
		NR (Poland)	NR	NR	0.8	CS = 5.0
		1979 (Sweden)	NR	NR	0.3	CS = 11.7
		1978 (U.K.	NR	NR	13.3	CS = 7.3
		1978 (Scotland)	NR	NR	13.0	CS = 10.7

Table 2.6.—*continued*

Reference	Type of Forceps	Years of Study (Country)	Total Deliveries	Forceps Deliveries	Incidence Forceps (%)	Comparison Figures (%)
Healy & Laufe (37)	All	1968 (U.S.)	NR	NR	29.7	CS = 5.5 (1970)
		1978 (U.S.)	NR	NR	12.2	CS = 15.2
Cosgrove et al. (28)	Low	NR (U.S.)	52,631	7,316	13.9	CS = 3.6

[a]VE, vacuum extraction delivery, unspecified instrument (almost exclusively the Malmström device); CS, cesarean section delivery; NR, not reported.

fetal tachycardia (>160 beats per minute (bpm)) or bradycardia (≤100 bpm). In the electronic fetal monitoring era, distress is more commonly diagnosed from a combination of observations including but not limited to the presence of meconium, an abnormal fetal heart rate tracing, and fetal scalp sampling data indicating acidosis/abnormal base deficit. Substantial judgment is necessary as cesarean delivery is often the best choice *unless* delivery can be promptly achieved from below with minimal maternal/fetal trauma (Table 2.3).

Cranial Malpresentation

Positioning of the presenting part often results in dystocia. This is especially true for deflection attitudes of the fetal head and asynclitism. When the fetal head is progressively deflexed, increasingly larger diameters are presented to the maternal pelvis (Figs. 2.18 and 2.19). This process results in either failure of the fetal head to

Table 2.7. Use of Assisted Delivery in Fetal Distress

Author	N	Technique	FD[a] (%)	Comments
Healy (39)	552	Midforceps	21	Kielland forceps
	95	Midforceps, with rotation	15	Non-Kielland forceps
	160	Manual rotation, forceps delivery	21	
Marin (40)	828	Midforceps	27.4	"mid cavity" with Barton forceps
Cosgrove (28)	1000	Midforceps, unspecified	7.1	FHR ≥160, ≤100 bpm were criteria for distress[b]
Chiswick & James (41)	86	Midforceps, Kielland's	19	"Fetal asphyxia"
Vacca (42)	152	Mid and low forceps, unspecified	19.7	Haig-Fergusson and Kielland forceps
Lasbrey (43)		Unspecified, forceps	44	

[a]FD, percent of forceps deliveries performed for the clinical diagnosis of fetal distress.
[b]FHR, fetal heart rate; bpm, beats per minute.

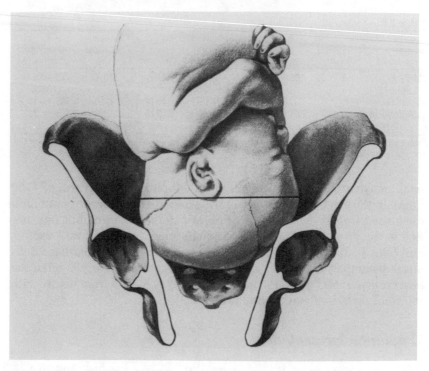

Figure 2.18.   Midposition (military or unflexed) fetal head. Note that the occipitofrontal diameter is presented to the pelvic inlet and engagement has not occurred. (From Bunn E. Grundriss zum studium der geburtshilfe. Muchen und Wiesbaden: Verlag von JF Bergman, 1922:576–577.)

enter the maternal pelvis or midpelvic arrest of progress and is unlikely to be overcome spontaneously.

Breech Presentation: Aftercoming Head

In breech presentation, the aim of the accoucheur is to maintain flexion of the fetal head and avoid dystocia either from malpresentation of the extremities (nuchal arms) or cranial entrapment (incomplete cervical dilatation or cranial deflection) (14, 44, 45). There is reasonable evidence that the routine application of forceps to the aftercoming head in breech presentation reduces fetal/neonatal injury (46). Forceps assistance is presumed to be beneficial for two major reasons: first, with the use of forceps, traction is not applied to the fetal shoulders or neck but to the skull itself, and second, the forceps may protect against decompression injuries occurring with uncontrolled crowning of the head.

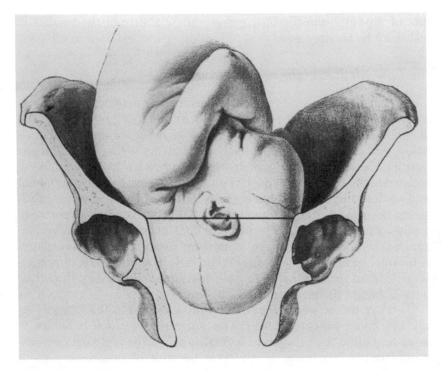

Figure 2.19. Well-flexed head. In comparison to Fig. 2.18, note how the suboccipitobregmatic diameter is now presented to the birth canal and the fetal head is engaged. (From Bunn E. Grundriss zum studium der gerburtshilfe. Muchen und Wiesbaden: Verlag von JF Bergman, 1922:576–577.)

Trial of Vaginal Delivery

A limited but important application for forceps is in a trial of vaginal birth when progress has arrested and the outcome is uncertain (see "Trial versus Failed Forceps"). The vacuum extractor also has an important role in trials of instrumental delivery (see Chapter 6).

Maternal Indications

Assisted delivery is sometimes required due simply to maternal exhaustion. A prolonged labor, large infant, limited maternal reserve, or a combination of these can necessitate assistance.

Uncommonly, special maternal conditions such as heart disease or intracranial lesions contraindicate Valsalva's maneuvers in the second stage and assisted delivery is indicated. Finally, under the effects of epidural anesthesia the urge and/or ability of the mother to push may be so attenuated that use of forceps is also required.

The Low Birth Weight or Premature Infant

For decades, since DeLee first voiced the concept of prophylactic forceps in the 1920s, the elective use of forceps in the delivery of the premature neonate has been practiced without serious critical evaluation. The "helmet" concept of assisted delivery is that use of forceps controls the expulsion of the premature fetal head. It is argued that the rigid protective case or helmet of the blades cushions the soft fetal head against the compressive forceps of second stage of labor, minimizing the risk(s) of intracranial injury (38). Intracranial hemorrhage in premature infants is a complex and controversial subject. The majority of hemorrhages in such premature infants are not associated with direct trauma but have more to do with complications of prematurity. It is uncertain what the role of instrumental delivery should be in the obstetric management of such cases (47, 48).

Any infant weight less than 1500 g falls into the category of very low birth weight (VLBW). The prognosis for such neonates is dependent upon their anatomic normality as well as perinatal management. Usually, an infant is ≤1500 g because of prematurity (≤32 weeks). Such infants are at gestational age (AGA) for their size. However, an infant can also be growth-retarded or small for gestational age (SGA) with a low birth weight confusing the analysis of such cases. All such VLBW neonates are particularly susceptible to asphyxia and/or traumatic injury (49). A major risk in such infants is intracranial hemorrhage, usually peri- or intraventricular (50).

Periventricular-intraventricular hemorrhage is the most common form of neonatal cerebral hemorrhage (51). This disorder is observed almost exclusively in newborns of <35 weeks and principally in those ≤32 weeks of gestational age (52). Its etiology is complex. Neonatal variables known to be associated with hemorrhages include low Apgar scores, gestational age (≤32 weeks), low birth weight, respiratory distress, pneumothorax, and metabolic imbalance (53, 54). Hemostasis abnormalities are common in neonates with hemorrhages but are not felt to be causal. Replacement or augmentation of such clotting factors does not prevent intracranial hemorrhages. However, recent evidence suggests a beneficial effect of ethamsylate (diethylammonia 2,5-dihydroxybenzene sulfonate) (54), a drug principally used in Europe to limit capillary bleeding in surgery. This agent is thought to affect platelet adhesiveness by modification of prostaglandin biosynthesis.

Real time ultrasonic scanning and computed axial tomography studies of the neonatal brain reveal that 20–50% of infants less than 1500 g have some degree of intracranial hemorrhage (52, 53). Only one-half of these cases can be diagnosed by unaided physical examination. Clinical signs and symptoms of hemorrhage vary from rapid neurologic deterioration to apparent normality (52, 55). The extent of hemorrhage and neonatal prognosis are closely related (55, 56). Fifty percent of periventricular and intraventricular hemorrhages occur in the first 24 hours of life. The remainder occur predominately within the following 48 hours. Such bleeds are strongly associated with complications of prematurity and its therapy (57). Extension in size of initial hemorrhages occurs after delivery, emphasizing the importance of serial scanning (56, 58). One-half of germinal matrix, two-thirds of intraventricular, and more than three-fourths of intracerebral hemorrhages occur more than 12 hours postpartum. Early neonatal events are of great importance in the development of bleeding (59). Alternatively, these same data have been used to argue that intrapartum events predispose to hemorrhages which then are diagnosed postnatally (60).

Pooled data (Table 2.8) indicate that long-term neurodevelopmental abnormalities are related to the extent of hemorrhage. Hemorrhage restricted to the germinal matrix has the best outcome while frank intracerebral hemorrhages carry the worst prognosis. The subsequent findings of persistent ventricular dilatation implying brain atrophy is an additional ominous sign, associated with both developmental delay and cerebral palsy (61, 62). Based on gross and microscopic data Wigglesworth (63) believes hemorrhages occur due to disruption of microcirculation within the germinal matrix. Disordered blood flow or hypoxia results in bleeding from the rupture of small capillaries within the subependymal germinal matrix over the lower part of the head of the caudate nucleus, directly opposite the foramen of Monro (63). In markedly premature infants (≤28 weeks), bleeding occurs at the level of the caudate nucleus, and in mature infants from the choroid plexus (63). In 80% of cases the hemorrhage extends into the ventricular system. Obliterative arachnoiditis is a common complication of such intraventrical blood (52). Porencephalic cysts from bleeding into the cerebral parenchyma or hydrocephalus are the unfortunate sequelae of these injuries. Possibly, transient rises of arterial pressure associated with neonatal apnea, accentuated by the cerebral vasodilation resulting from asphyxia associated with respiratory distress syndrome (RDS) are etiologic. Increases in arterial pressure in premature neonates are believed to be especially dangerous, as they produce greater increases in transmural pressure in the brain of the premature than occur in full-term neonates. Studies of cerebral blood flow in

Table 2.8. Risk of Long Term Neurodevelopmental Damage from Neonatal Periventricular Hemorrhage[a]

Ultrasound Findings	No. of Survivors	No. (%) with Morbidity	Range of Morbidity (%)
No periventricular hemorrhage	678	63 (9)	4–27
Germinal matrix hemorrhage	199	40 (20)	9–50
Intraventricular hemorrhage	150	61 (41)	29–67
Intracerebral hemorrhage	83	71 (86)	50–100

[a]Pooled data from 11 centers. Modified from Szymonowicz W, Yu VYH, Bajuk B, Astbury J. Neurodevelopmental outcome of periventricular haemorrhage and leukomalacia in infants 1250 g or less at birth. Early Hum Dev. 1986; 14:1–7.

infants with respiratory distress syndrome document *increased* cerebral flow preceeding hemorrhage and, paradoxically, *decreased* flow in asphyxiated neonates (64, 65). In animal models induction of either hypertension or hypercapnia results in intraventricular hemorrhages. In asphyxiated full-term neonates, fetal scalp asphyxia also increases blood flow in deep cerebral structures (66). The neonatal brain thus has difficulty in autoregulation of its blood flow (52). Particularly important are factors that *increase* the pressure gradient between the blood vessel lumen in the germinal matrix and the surrounding brain tissues. Blood flow to the critical periventricular region is markedly sensitive to fluctuations in arterial blood pressure. The initiating event in subependymal or germinal matrix hemorrhage is probably either hyper- or hypoperfusion of the brain. Initial rises in arterial pressure with hypercapnia/apnea or possibly with cranial distortion (e.g., forceps, vacuum extraction, entrapped head) or restoration of flow to an ischemic brain (e.g., secondary to hypotension, hypoxia) disrupts the subependymal germinal matrix microcirculation and hemorrhage results (63).

The preterm brain is anatomically predisposed to hemorrhage. A relatively large proportion of total cerebral blood flow is directed to the basal ganglia and subependymal maxtrix regions. Further, the vascular channels within the matrix consist of an irregular rete system—not mature capillaries. Thus a system exists with immature bridging vessels lying deep within the fetal brain in an area receiving a disproportionate amount of the total cerebral blood flow (52, 63).

The sum of the clinical evidence indicates that prevention of respiratory distress and its accompanying asphyxia and, to a lesser degree, avoidance of perinatal trauma will reduce the risk of periventricular hemorrhages. Hypoxia, hypercapnia, hypovolemia, hypotension, assisted ventilation, and physiologic trauma during delivery are the critical contributing perinatal factors. Based on both neonatal ultrasound data and necropsy findings Tejani (67) proposes that periventricular hemorrhage begins in the antepartum period and is the *cause* rather than the *result* of premature labor. If true, methods of delivery have only a limited relationship to the incidence of neonatal hemorrhage. In the search for data to support this hypothesis, the effects of mode of delivery are unclear. Some reviews conclude that the method of delivery is not associated or weakly associated with the risk of hemorrhage (46, 53, 67, 68, 69, 70, 71, 72, 73, 74), while others report an apparent protective effect of either cesarean delivery (49, 75, 76) or forceps use (33, 77, 78, 79, 80) or a protective effect only under certain circumstances (81). Others such as O'Driscoll (82) believe that prophylactic forceps actually increase the risk of intracranial hemorrhage and should be abandoned. *It appears that the critical factor is the extent or degree of birth injury from whatever cause and not specifically the mode of delivery.* A difficult cesarean delivery of an already asphyxiated fetus may well be more dangerous than a carefully controlled vaginal delivery with or without forceps (see Chapter 6).

Contraindications to Forceps Use

The contraindications to forceps use fall into several categories (Table 2.9): *inexperience with the various instruments and/or techniques, inadequate trial of labor,* and *uncertainty of fetal position.* No instrumental delivery should be attempted if the intention is to overcome cephalopelvic disproportion. Cesarean section is the correct management in such circumstances (see also Tables 2.3 and 2.5).

Failure of Instrumental Delivery

Instrumental delivery is not invariably successful. While practitioners of even mediocre skill can adequately perform cesarean delivery, the appropriate use of instruments in vaginal delivery requires substantially greater experience, skill and judgment. An important but commonly ignored issue in instrumental vaginal delivery is the human factor. Nothing can substitute for experience, long practice, and *sang-*

Table 2.9.   Contraindications to Forceps Use

Uncertainty of fetal position/station
Inadequate anesthesia/analgesia
Operator inexperience
True cephalopelvic disproportion
Inadequate trial of labor
Undilated cervix

froid in an accoucheur. The practitioner must assess the course in labor, fetal condition, and the anatomy of the patient and determine if further uterine stimulation, maternal repositioning, administration of anesthesia, or cesarean delivery are better alternatives to an attempt at instrumental delivery. A measure of humility is also required as clinical impressions are not invariably accurate even when rendered by the most careful practitioner.

If assisted delivery is chosen but fails, it is important to question the circumstances. In general, failure to deliver from below by forceps or vacuum is due either to a *failure in the initial application* of the chosen instrument or a *failure in extraction* once the instrument has been correctly applied. Errors in clinical judgment, lack of sufficient skill, or unforeseen difficulties contribute to both categories of failure.

Application Failure

Incomplete Dilatation

If the cervix is not fully dilated, the forceps blades are difficult or impossible to correctly insert (83). If forceps blades are inserted through the cervix, dystocia can result as forceps traction is partially overcoming cervical resistance. *Thus, incomplete dilatation is a contraindication to forceps application and a relative contraindication to an attempt at vacuum extraction.* Cesarean delivery is usually the best choice if the cervix is found to be incompletely dilated unless the labor can be prolonged. Manual cervical dilatation, unless of minimal extent in multiparas, usually results in cervical laceration and is to be avoided.

Position of the Fetal Head

The process of labor on the fetal head normally results in cranial molding and formation of scalp edema. Following dystotic labor, it can become impossible to insert blades or to be certain of the accuracy of their application. The combination of molding and caput succedaneum formation can so obscure landmarks that even an experienced clinician has difficulty in assessing fetal position. Careful attention to palpation of the cranial fontanelles and the suture lines, and the orbital ridges if deflection exists, usually establishes the correct cranial orientation. In uncertain cases, if good epidural anesthesia is present, the operator can also palpate for the fetal ear, taking care not to displace the fetal head. On occasion, real time ultrasound is helpful, particularly in occiput posterior positions, in localizing the fetal orbits or other cranial anatomy. Occasionally, the vacuum extractor can be applied in the setting of uncertain landmarks as the location of the cup on the fetal head is less critical than the orientation of the forceps blades. However, even with the vacuum extractor accurate localization of at least the occiput is required (see Chapter 4). In all cases, when the fetal head is markedly molded, disproportion must be carefully considered before any application is attempted or traction is applied. Leopold's maneuvers and careful suprapubic palpation will exclude some cases from trial by noting a high cephalic part or by suggesting fetal macrosomia. There is no modern indication for x-ray pelvimetry in establishing either fetal station or position.

It is particularly in the setting of a heavily molded and edematous fetal head that greatest care in assisted delivery is required. The observation of marked molding and caput proves that the cephalopelvic relationship is tight. The use of forceps or the vacuum extractor to overcome true disproportion is inappropriate and potentially dangerous to both mother and child. The desire for vaginal delivery is not to be interpreted as a physical struggle where force overcomes both anatomic obstruction and prudence. In *accouchement forcé*, when unyielding steel instruments are inserted into a bony canal of fixed dimensions, the victor will always be the attendant but the costs are paid by the mother and child.

Extraction Failure

In failure of extraction an instrument is correctly applied, traction is initiated, but delivery does not occur. This is the setting where the greatest clinical experience and self control for the clinician must be exercised (see discussion on "Trial versus Failed Forceps"). Reasons for unsuccessful extraction are as follows.

Malposition/Malpresentation

If the fetal head is presenting into the pelvis without complete flexion, a larger diameter faces the birth canal (Figs. 2.18 and 2.19) (84). As the fetal head progressively deflexes through the military position toward the brow, the largest diameter of the fetal head increases from approximately 9 cm (suboccipital-bregmatic) to 12.5 cm (occipitomental) (see Fig. 4.3). Failure to observe and correct deflection results in a difficult or impossible accouchement. Occiput posterior positions are also commonly associated with dystocia, due in part to cranial deflection (85).

Cephalopelvic or Fetopelvic Disproportion

Failure to extract the fetus can be due simply to excessive fetal size (macrosomia). The incidence of midpelvic delivery rises substantially when fetal weight exceeds 4000 g. Relative fetopelvic disproportion can also occur. The pelvic architecture may be gynecoid in shape or adequate by measurement but still associated with dystocia. This can be due to a large fetus in a relatively small pelvis, partial deflection of the fetal head, and/or incoordinate uterine activity and asynclitism. Uncommonly, fetal tumors arising from the head or neck (cystic hygromas, enlarged thyroid, hydrocephaly, teratomas, etc.), conjoined twins, twins in collision, maternal tumor, or other pelvic masses also produce obstruction sufficient to prevent delivery from below.

The estimation of fetal weight by simple abdominal palpation is fraught with error. The best correlate with baby size is *maternal size*. Unfortunately, it is precisely in the larger patient, where fetal size estimation is most critical, that maternal bulk makes the determination most difficult. Fetal size can often be reasonably estimated by ultrasound nomograms, using either the biparietal diameter or femur length and the abdominal circumference as the major parameters (86, 87). The relationship between the abdominal and biparietal diameters (BPD) is also helpful in judging the risk for shoulder girdle dystocia. If the BPD-abdominal diameter difference exceeds 1.4 cm, dystocia is more likely, but not certain (88, 89).

Constriction Ring and Pathologic Retraction Ring (Bandl's Ring)

Retraction rings of the uterus are an uncommon but dramatic cause of dystocia (90). A pathologic retraction ring (Bandl's ring) develops at the division between the upper, contractile segment of the uterus and the lower, nonmuscular portion. The fetal shoulders/thorax are blocked from further descent by the ring, rendering delivery per vagina impossible. On occasion, such rings are so tight that delivery is difficult even with cesarean section. A peculiar "figure 8" shape of the lower uterine segment in a thin patient with dystotic labor suggests the correct diagnosis. Cesarean section is the appropriate method of delivery in this situation. Unless the ring is surgically incised or the uterus relaxed by the administration of tocolytics or halgonated inhalation agents, extraction by abdominal delivery can still be difficult.

The pathologic retraction ring is not to be confused with a constriction ring (90). Constriction rings are thought to be the *result* of localized uterine irritability. Such rings grip the fetus and prevent its descent. In contradistinction to pathologic retraction rings, constriction rings occur in any portion of the uterus. A constriction ring usually forms in an irritable uterus following desultory labor, especially if intrauterine manipulations have been performed or oxytocin administered (20).

Bandl's ring—the true pathologic retraction ring—forms as a *result* of obstructed labor. The lower uterine segment is tense and often tender to palpation, progress is poor, and the labor usually prolonged. Uterine rupture may occur if delivery by cesarean section is not promptly performed. In contrast, constriction rings are the *cause* of obstructed labor and are much less ominous. Management in the latter case may be uterine relaxation, stopping of oxytocin stimulation, or cesarean section if progress has been poor.

Problems of Fetal Station

Excessive molding of the fetal head, accompanied by formation of scalp edema (caput succedaneum), occasionally results in a situation where the apparent presenting part is at or near the perineum but when the true biparietal diameter is at a much higher station (Fig. 2.20). Application of forceps or vacuum initially appears easy, but with traction no station is made. When such cases are taken to cesarean delivery, extraction of the fetal head from above can be ex-

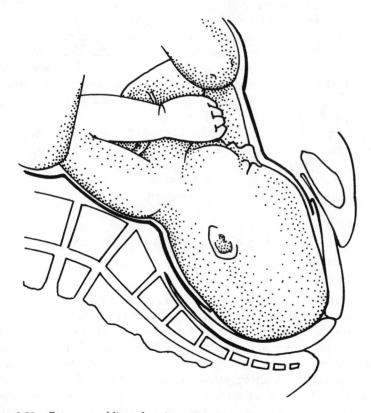

Figure 2.20. Extreme molding of occiput posterior presentation. Note caput reaching the perineum but high station of the biparietal diameter of the fetal head. (After Dennon EH. Forceps deliveries. 2nd ed. Philadelphia: FA Davis, 1964.)

tremely difficult or traumatic to the lower uterine segment unless the head is elevated *per vagina* by direct upward pressure provided by an assistant stationed below the operative drapes.

Poor Obstetrical Judgment

On occasion, forceps may be applied when the cervix is incompletely dilated or unrecognized deflection or asynclitism is present. Traction either results in failure and/or cervical laceration.

The most serious problem occurs when blades or the vacuum are applied, and when dystocia is clearly present, but the accoucheur is determined to achieve delivery from below regardless of difficulty. Despite heroics, vaginal delivery may, in fact, not occur. In a struggle between an adult with unyielding metal blades working within a fixed, bony enclosure on a fetus with a compressible cranium, the ultimate victor is obvious. The expense of such folly is, of course, borne by the fetus. Maternal injuries in such a debacle are also common and occasionally severe. It is not simply the inexperienced who are occasionally trapped in this dismal scenario. With application of the blades and firm traction, fetal head compression occurs, commonly accompanied by bradycardia. Here the clinician is also trapped. Now it appears that fetal distress has supervened and the accoucheur redoubles his/her efforts. Some parctitioners simply cannot stop and reassess, perhaps even displacing the fetal head upward before proceeding to cesarean delivery. Clinical judgment is not an exact science and a dogmatic approach to assisted vaginal delivery is fraught with maternal and fetal danger. Surgeons must always recall that *all forceps and vacuum extractor operations are to some extent trials. Accouchement forcé* performed to please the obstetrician is never acceptable.

Trial versus Failed Forceps and Trial versus Failed Vacuum Extraction

It is important to distinguish in our thinking between a *trial of forceps* or vacuum extraction and *failed forceps or vacuum extraction*. Unfortunately, in recent literature, these procedures are often discussed as synonymous. In a *trial* the operator has decided that further attempts at vaginal delivery by stimulation of uterine activity, repositioning the patient, waiting, etc. are not likely to be efficacious or there is evidence of a fetal or maternal problem that necessitates prompt delivery. *The operator is prepared for immediate cesarean section if the forceps or vacuum extraction delivery is not successful.* Forceps or vacuum application is attempted. If application is successful, traction is applied. If no descent occurs, the procedure is abandoned and the patient is promptly delivered by cesarean section. Such trials require a most careful and experienced clinician and the judicious application of force. *Trial of forceps* or *vacuum extraction* remains a perfectly appropriate obstetrical procedure, albeit with carefully limited indications.

The term *failed forceps* or *failed vacuum extraction* is re-served for cases in which *forceps or the vacuum extractor are applied with the anticipation of delivery from below but fail, with or without trauma to the mother and/or fetus.* In this scenario, the attempt has not been accompanied by preparations for alternative delivery. A failed procedure implies that the operator has misjudged the extent of dys-tocia and that true disproportion exists (91, 92).

All attempts at instrumental vaginal delivery are, in fact, trials. Judgment is necessary in deciding how extensive an effort is appropri-ate. One of the difficulties in making the distinction between trial and failed forceps or vacuum extraction retrospectively by record review is that, without careful reading of the operative note, it can be impossible to determine which procedure was intended. The distinction between these procedures is not academic. In the one, the operator begins with the realization that the outcome is uncertain and he/she is prepared for prompt operative intervention following a judicious application of force. In the second case, the possibility of failure is not seriously entertained in advance and neither the patient nor the operator is nec-essarily prepared for the likelihood of failure.

What are the risks to a trial of instrumental delivery? If the costs to failed or trial forceps were serious maternal or fetal injury, we could never countenance the attempt. In our consideration of risks, the fetal and maternal results of failed procedures need to be compared against the outcome of successful midpelvic delivery by forceps/vac-uum or cesarean section. These are the options open to the obstetrician when dystocia or fetal distress is present and spontaneous delivery not anticipated.

It is difficult to research the issue of maternal-fetal risk from trials versus failed forceps and little data are available for vacuum extraction (Table 2.10). Further, most series cannot separate trials of delivery from traumatic failed forceps. Especially in older literature, the failed forceps procedures described include high forceps and other heroic procedures in which the attempt was to avoid cesarean delivery at all costs. Data available from the contemporary studies of Hughey and coworkers (98), Cardozo et al. (26), and Boyd et al. (92) are helpful. The incidence of failed procedures varies from 1.10 to 6.1%. These data are somewhat misleading and not entirely comparable, as the au-

Table 2.10. Failed Forceps, Selected Series

Author	No. of Instrumental Vaginal Deliveries Attempted	No. of Failed Procedures	% Fetal Morbidity	Fetal Mortality	Maternal Morbidity	Maternal Mortality
Murray (93)		52		31/52 (59.6%)[a]		8/52 (15.4%)
Miller (94)	500	88 (17.8%)		46/88 (52.3%)	39/88 (44.3%)	17/88 (19%)
Claye (95)		49		38/49 (77.6%)	19/49 (38.7%)	4/49 (8.2%)
Freeth (96)		100		30/92[b] (33%)[c]	5/100 (5%)	2/100 (2%)
Law (97)		37		7.36 (22.2%)	19.37 (27%)	0
Decker et al. (27)	547	9 Midforceps (1.6%)		4/9 (44%)		0
Hughey et al. (98)	9317 Low forceps 1570 Mid-forceps	18 (0.16%)	3/18[d] (17%)	0	8/18 (44%)	0
Cardozo et al. (26)	297 Primipara	18 (6.1%)		0		0
	59 Multipara	2 (3.4%)		0		0
Boyd et al. (92)	2353 Low forceps 1276 Mid-forceps	53 (0.8%)[e]	13/53 (24.5%)[f]	0		0

[a] 23 of 31 (74%) were dead *in utero* on admission.
[b] 8 of 100 (8%) were dead *in utero* on admission.
[c] 6/8 were dead *in utero* on admission.
[d] 5 minute Apgar <7.
[e] Total, 4% for midforceps.
[f] Neonatal intensive care unit (NICU) admissions, in comparison, in cases of cesarean section for failure to progress, 23.2% of neonates were also NICU admissions, a nonsignificant difference (see also Table 2.12).

thors vary in the presentation of their data. In general, patients requiring either forceps assistance or cesarean section are more likely to have undergone induction, experienced longer labors, or shown signs of fetal distress (Table 2.11). The most appropriate comparison group for the morbidity/mortality of failed forceps procedures is first, cases of women taken to cesarean section for failure to progress/dystocia and secondly, instances of successful midforceps delivery. When these groups are chosen, outcome results are generally comparable (Table 2.12).

In sum, either a "trial of forceps" or a "trial of vacuum extraction" is an acceptable obstetric procedure. "Failed forceps" or "failed vacuum extraction" implies a failure in clinical judgment. Such failures occur uncommonly even to experienced accoucheurs. However, in a correctly conducted trial *neither fetal nor maternal injury should occur.* It is well to recall Stacey (99), who commented in reference to failed/trial forceps that ". . . it is certain that of all the aids we possess in the safe delivery of women in labour, none is of greater value than the practice of the art of patience."

Trial of Instrumental Delivery: Clinical Setting

Failure of Progress or Fetal Distress

The accoucheur must carefully consider the fetal condition. If the electronic monitoring tracing indicates distress, the choice of delivery route will need to be made with dispatch. If full dilatation is present and the head is at +1 or greater, vacuum extraction or, on occasion, a prompt forceps application can achieve delivery more rapidly than cesarean section. If progress has failed and no immediate fetal danger is present, then the multiple considerations previously reviewed can be considered with more leisure (molding, possible cranial deflection, macrosomia, etc.) in reaching a conclusion as to how to proceed.

Procedure

The forceps blades or the vacuum cup are applied. Moderate traction is produced during contractions with release of tension between attempts. If delivery is not achieved following a maximum of five pulls with progress beginning with the *initial* traction effort, the procedure is abandoned and cesarean section performed. It is to be emphasized that *descent should be apparent with the first traction,* if not, the most careful reassessment is required.

Anesthesia

Trials are best attempted with epidural anesthesia. Thus, if the accouchement is unsuccessful, operative delivery can proceed from above with dispatch. Occasionally, forceps can be attempted under pudendal block but the application/traction or a midpelvic trial may be distressing to the patient and this approach is not recommended. Vacuum extraction can in general be attempted with less anesthesia than forceps and trials under pudendal block are often reasonable (see

Table 2.11. Characteristics of Labor by Method of Delivery[a]

	No. of Cases	Induction (%)	Duration (h)	Prolonged[b] (%)	Abnormal Fetal Heart (%)	Meconium in Amniotic Fluid (%)
Spontaneous	2760	12.7	9.6	9.6	11.1	15.6
Low forceps	2353	17.8[c]	10.5[c]	10.1	19.5[c]	16.8
Midforceps	1276	16.9[c]	11.3[c]	14.0[c]	33.6[c]	22.1[c]
CS with failure to progress	82	13.4	13.8[c]	24.6[c]	33.3[c]	29.3[c]
CS with failed forceps	53	20.8	13.5[c]	17.8	34.0[c]	26.4[c]

[a]CS, cesarean section. From Boyd ME, Usher RH, McLean FH, Normal BE. Failed forceps. Obstet Gynecol 1986; 68:779–783.
[b]Prolonged labor defined as greater than 18 hours.
[c]$P < 0.05$, as compared with spontaneous deliveries.

Chapter 4). Saddle block anesthesia can be used in either setting, but if the effort fails, a second anesthetic is required for cesarean delivery.

Personnel, Setting

Ideally, trials should occur in the operating room with an anesthesiologist, nurses, and an operative assistant present. Thus, no time will be lost in collecting personnel and equipment if cesarean delivery is required.

Table 2.12. Outcome by Method of Delivery[a]

	No. of Cases	Depression at Birth (%) Moderate	Depression at Birth (%) Severe	Enceph-alopathy (%)	Meconium Aspiration (%)	Fractures or Palsies (%)	Admission to NICU[b] (%)
Spontaneous	2760	2.0	0.3	0.1	0.4	0.6	7.9
Low forceps	2353	1.7	0.3	0.1	0.3	1.2[c]	8.7
Midforceps	1276	4.0[c]	0.3	0.4	0.4	5.1[c]	18.8[c]
CS for failure to progress	82	11.0[c]	2.4[c]	2.4[c]	2.4	0.0	23.2[c, d]
CS after failed forceps	53	11.3[c]	1.9	5.7[c]	3.8[c]	3.8[c]	24.5[c, d]

[a]From Boyd ME, Usher RH, McLean FH, Normal BE. Failed forceps. Obstet Gynecol 1986; 68:779–783.
[b]NICU, neonatal intensive care unit.
[c]$P < 0.05$ as compared with spontaneous deliveries.
[d]Not significantly different.

Table 2.13. Factors Predictive of Forceps Use

Nulliparity
Maternal height/weight
Abnormalities of labor
Birth weight > 4000 g
Epidural anesthesia

Forceps Use: Clinical Associations

The need for assisted delivery is generally predictable (Table 2.13). Larger mothers and babies, administration of anesthesia, nulliparity, and abnormalities of labor all increase the likelihood of instrumental delivery.

Parity

Virtually all studies observe an association between nulliparity and the use of forceps (Table 2.14). Not surprisingly, labors in women with an untested pelvis are more likely to require assistance than parturitions occurring among multiparas.

Maternal Height

Shorter mothers appear to more commonly require delivery assistance. Chiswick and James (41) studied 86 babies delivered with Kielland forceps compared to 86 spontaneous vaginal deliveries. These pregnancies were matched for maternal age, parity, and whether labor was induced or spontaneous. They found that the mean maternal

Table 2.14. Nulliparity and the Use of Forceps

Reference	No. in Series	Type of Forceps Delivery	Nulliparous (%)
Taylor (100)	31	Mid	74
Cosgrove & Weaver (28)	1000	Mid	68
Lasbrey et al. (43)	131	All, unspecified	67
Cooke (23)	427	Mid	62
Dunlop (32)	292	Mid	62
Marin (40)	248	Mid Barton forceps	83
Chiswick & James (41)	86	Kielland	75.6
Bowes & Bowes (33)	71	Mid	80
Healy et al. (39)	552	Kielland for rotation and delivery	71
Vacca et al. (42)	152	All, unspecified	90
Cardozo et al. (26)	336	Nonrotational, ventouse, Kielland	83
Benkus et al. (101)	84	All	64

height was significantly less in the Kielland-delivered group. Further, the mean ratio of maternal height to neonatal occipitofrontal head circumference was significantly smaller in the women requiring forceps delivery than in the control group. In contrast, Cardozo et al. (26) failed to observe an association between maternal height and the use of forceps in primigravidas or multigravidas. The association between maternal size is complex and relates more to total maternal bulk than simply height along. Baby size is best predicted by maternal size. Thus short, obese women are at a disadvantage for dystocia.

Abnormalities of Labor

Various abnormalities in the course of labor are associated with a higher likelihood of instrumental delivery. Failure to progress for a combination of reasons is by far the most common difficulty (Table 2.15). For example, Chiswick and James (41) found the interval between engagement of the fetal head and onset of labor longer in patients who required midforceps versus those with spontaneous vaginal deliveries. This difference was maintained even when primiparous and multiparous women were considered separately. The rate of cervical dilatation is also important. Among nulliparas the mean time for the cervix to dilate from 4 to 7 cm is significantly longer among cases eventually delivered using Kielland forceps than those with spontaneous delivery. Further, among both nulliparas and multiparas the mean time for the cervix to dilate from 7 to 10 cm is significantly longer among cases where Kielland forceps were used than among women

Table 2.15.   Factors Predisposing to Second Stage Failure to Progress[a]

Relative uterine inertia
  Spontaneous uncoordinate uterine activity
  Inadequate stimulation
Relative cephalopelvic disproportion/obstruction
  Fetal malpresentation (OP, extension) face, brow[b]
  Fetal macrosomia
  Pelvic inadequacy (android, platypelloid type)
  Rigid perineum or cervix
  Obstructed outlet
    Twins in collision
    Fetal/maternal tumor
  Formation of pathologic retraction ring (Bandl's ring)
Other factors
  Epidural anesthesia inhibiting normal rotation
  Maternal exhaustion/debility
  Improper positioning, inadequate coaching or encouragement

[a]Modified from Oxorn H. Human labor and birth. 4th ed. New York: Appleton-Century-Crofts, 1980.
[b]OP, occiput posterior.

experiencing spontaneous deliveries. Cooke (23), in a study of 427 midforceps deliveries from 1960 to 1965, observed that 89% were performed for the primary indication of midpelvic arrest and a further 5.8% were performed for the primary indication of combined midpelvic arrest and fetal distress.

Malposition/Malpresentation

Not surprisingly, abnormalities of fetal positioning are associated with dystocia and the requirement for instrumental assistance (31) (Table 2.16). Cosgrove and Weaver (28) observed that, among 1000 midforceps, 67% were performed for the primary indication of dystocia, which they defined as deep pelvic arrest or inertia. Finally, Taylor (100) in a review of 31 midforceps deliveries, recorded that 81% were performed for the primary indication of uterine inertia, associated with delayed second stage with arrest of head at the midpelvis. Failure to negotiate the midpelvis due either to pelvic inadequacy or failure of powers is the predominate reason for instrumental delivery (102).

Prolonged Second Stage of Labor

Delayed progress in expulsion of the fetus is a common indication for the use of forceps, especially midforceps (103). However, the definition of "prolonged" for the second stage of labor is not firmly established (Table 2.17). Many authors establish different time periods for multiparas versus nulliparas. Depending upon the study, the sec-

Table 2.16. Association between Forceps Use and Fetal Malpresentation

Author	N	Procedure	Fetal Position	Forceps use (%) Indication for this
Healy et al. (39)	95	Rotation and delivery (non-Kielland)	OP[a]	16
			LOP, ROP	62
Healy et al. (39)	160	Manual rotation, unspecified forceps	OP	31
			LOP, ROP	45
Marin (40)	248	Barton	OP, oblique	9.3
			OP	
			OT[b]	90.7
Dunlop (32)	292	Unspecified	OA	36.7
		Midforceps	OT	26.4
			OP	35.9
			Unspecified	1.0

[a]OP, occiput posterior; LOP, left occiput posterior; ROP, right occiput posterior; OA, occiput anterior; OT, occiput transverse.
[b]Or "near transverse."

Table 2.17. Prolonged Second Stage and Forceps Use

Author	N	Procedure	PSS[a] (%)	Author's Definition PSS
Marin (40)	248	Midforceps Barton	60	>45 min nullipara, >30 min multipara
Bowes & Bowes (33)	71	Midforceps	56	>2 hours
Chiswick & James (41)	86	Midforceps Kielland	56	>60 min nullipara, >30 min multipara
Vacca et al. (42)	152	Mid and outlet Haig-Fergusson and Kielland	66[b]	Not specified
Schenker & Serr (104)	300	Unspecified forceps	28.3	Not specified
Healy et al. (39)	502	Midforceps Kielland	50 (OP) 27 (OT)	Not specified

[a]Prolonged second stage of labor; comparison to current recommendations (Table 2.5) is interesting.

ond stage for a nullipara has been described as prolonged if it exceeds 45 minutes to 2 hours. The corresponding range for multiparas is 30 to 60 minutes. Thus, wide latitude exists for the potential use of assisted delivery (see discussion under "Epidural Anesthesia"). Recent American College of Obstetricians and Gynecologists guidelines suggest that the second stage is prolonged in primigravidas if it exceeds 3 hours when a regional anesthetic has been given or more than 2 hours in the absence of regional anesthetic. The time limits for multiparas are more than 2 hours if a regional anesthetic has been administered and more than 1 hour if it has not (Table 2.5).

Fetal Macrosomia

There is a general trend toward increasing rates of instrumentation in progressively larger infants especially when fetal size exceeds 4000 g (23, 32, 42).

Epidural Anesthesia

It is generally held that epidural anesthesia increases the rate of fetal malposition and instrumentation by altering the second stage of labor (105–108). However, such has not been the finding by all observers. There is some evidence that the second stage is minimally affected if careful choice of agent and/or anesthetic technique occurs (109, 110). The increased likelihood of instrumental delivery following epidural anesthesia is due to several factors. Regional anesthesia can reduce the strength of uterine contractions (106, 111). Johnson and coworkers (106) recorded the pressure of spontaneous contractions as well as the contribution of maternal voluntary efforts in total force in patients before and after induction of conduction anesthesia with 1% lidocaine. In normal patients without conduction anesthesia, increases in voluntary effort occurred as the second stage progressed. In contrast, women with epidural blocks showed declines in the strength of spontaneous *and* voluntary efforts despite active coaching. However, these findings were not consistent in all cases. In some instances women actually exhibited an increased ability to bear down after receiving the conduction anesthetic, emphasizing the importance of individual variation.

Part of the delivery delay is due to anesthetic-induced changes in the tone of the pelvic musculature. The normal mechanism for fetal expulsion in the second stage of labor is complex. Passage of the fetus through the various planes of the pelvis occurs due to spontaneous uterine contractions aided by voluntary expulsive efforts of the mother. The mechanism of labor in the second stage is influenced by the shape of the fetal head, its flexion or deflection, and the architecture of the muscular and bony passages of the pelvis. In general, the fetal head takes the path of least resistance, driven by uterine activity. Rotation is governed by an interaction between the presenting part, the muscles of the lower pelvis (particularly the levator ani), and the shape of the bony pelvis; however, this relationship is not simple. If cranial rotation occurred solely as a result of the tone of the pelvic floor muscles, fetal malposition should occur in all patients with severe motor blockade, but this does not happen. Still, both instrumental delivery and severe motor block are more common in patients with the most profound analgesia.

There is also evidence indicating that lower pelvic sensory/motor blockade interferes with the physiology of uterine activity (111, 112). Spontaneous uterine contractions are believed to progressively increase in strength during the second stage of labor although this has never been directly demonstrated (111). Clinically, this corresponds to the transitional stage of labor where laboring women frequently perceive or report more intense contractions, usually rapidly followed a desire to bear down as the presenting part descends further within the birth canal. There is evidence from both animal and human experimentation suggesting that the increased strength of contractions in the second stage results from the release of oxytocin from the posterior lobe of the pituitary gland (113). Distention of the birth canal presumably stimulates sensory impulses that travel to the hypothalamus, resulting in oxytocin release (114, 115). In the 1940s, Ferguson (114) emphasized the importance of an intact nervous system in parturition when he demonstrated that increases in uterine activity brought about by dilatation of the birth canal in rabbits were abolished by cord transsection. In human labor, epidural analgesia, by blocking the pelvic autonomic nerves, can prevent or blunt the rise in oxytocin expected during the second stage. It is theorized that the small diameter of the pelvic parasympathetic nerves predisposes them to prolonged blockage (116). Thus, a neurohumeral reflex—similar to the Ferguson reflex—may exist that is partially blocked by anesthesia, especially dense anesthesia. This interference alters normal second stage physiology in many but not all labors.

Suggestive clinical evidence exists for epidural blockade and human labor, supporting the idea that blockade of a neurohumoral mechanism occurs in women given regional anesthesia. Overall uterine activity in the second stage of labor is reduced 15% in nulliparas and 20% in multiparas with epidural anesthesia when compared to normal controls (111). These data support augmentation of the second stage of labor with oxytocin in patients undergoing epidural anesthesia (117). In fact, if oxytocin is given in second stage labor, the incidence of forceps delivery declines substantially (117). Thus, the more profound the motor and sensory block, the greater the likelihood of abolishing the *reflex* urge to push as well as the patient's *ability* to push (108, 118). These effects are cumulative, resulting in delayed progress.

Based on these data it is not surprising that both the agents used and the techniques for managing pain relief in the second stage affect the likelihood of instrumental delivery (109–111, 118–120). Earlier studies on epidural anesthesia and instrumental delivery frequently employed lidocaine, which produces a dense motor and sensory block. More recent studies using bupivacaine (Marcaine) (118) show that using lower concentrations of this anesthetic agent, particularly the 0.25% concentration, results in both a higher incidence of spontaneous delivery and a reduction in the incidence of instrumental delivery with no change in cesarean section rate.

Anesthetic technique is also important in influencing the second stage and can be modified to achieve minimal disruption of the labor process based upon our understanding of how women perceive pain during labor (121). Labor pain or discomfort has both a uterine and perineal origin. Pain from the uterus is transmitted primarily through the XIth and XIIth thoracic spinal cord segments. In contrast, pain arising from the perineum, normally felt in the latter part of labor, is transmitted via the pelvic somatic nerves through the II, III, and IV sacral segments, which also provide the motor supply to the muscles of the pelvic floor (121). Modifications of epidural anesthetic technique aim to either selectively block higher segments early in labor and lower segments later, or to choose agents or methods of drug administration that less profoundly inhibit muscular tone in the attempt to preserve muscle strength such that, with voluntary bearing down, spontaneous rotation is more likely.

Obstetric management is also important. There have been a number of attempts to offset the effect of epidural analgesia by changing the dynamics of the second stage of labor. Repositioning, coaching, and administration of oxytocin are the common treatments (117, 122). It is best to rethink our definitions of prolonged second stage when epidural anesthesia has been given. Simple extension of the second stage of labor as long as progress is being made is not necessarily associated with any increase in perinatal morbidity or mortality as long as adequate fetal monitoring is performed (121). It is inappropriate to judge the length of the second stage of labor in patients with epidural anesthesia against norms developed for women who have labored without a regional block.

Other techniques to reduce the likelihood of instrumental delivery have been practiced with mixed results. Some practitioners have allowed epidural anesthesia to wear off in the second stage of labor under the belief that this will improve the patient's ability to push. This usually proves counterproductive. Phillips and Thomas (123) tested this proposal in two groups of women entering the second stage. In one the epidural block was allowed to wear off in the second stage of labor while in the second the analgesia was maintained throughout. Not surprisingly, the group with the anesthesia maintained experienced less pain but actually had *shorter* second stages in comparison to the group whose block was allowed to wear off. Further, the group with the continuous block did not on average require increased dosages of the analgesic drug. The rate of assisted or forceps delivery in women with continuous block was actually *lower* than in those where the block was allowed to wear off, and there were fewer instances of fetal distress and persisting malrotations. Thus, allowing the epidural anesthetic to wear off increases patient discomfort and dissatisfaction with the birth process but does not necessarily reduce the incidence of instrumental delivery when the second stage is appropriately managed. The rapid return of pain in a patient who has been essentially pain-free during the preceeding hours of labor probably results in the prompt elevation of plasma catecholamines, which interfere with myometrial function, contributing to dysfunctional labor.

Perhaps Crawford (124) is correct. He argues that current clinical management of the second stage is simply faulty, predicated on an arbitrary definition or lack of definition of the commencement of the second stage. Usually when full cervical dilatation has been identified by vaginal examination, the mother is urged to bear down whether she feels the need or not, even though the period of full cervical dilatation is never known with certainty unless continuous cervical examinations have been performed. Crawford believes that the mother should not be encouraged to bear down *unless she feels the urge to do so and full cervical dilatation is present, or until the presenting part is distending the perineum.* Further, if progress is being made and if there is no evidence of fetal distress or undue maternal fatigue, then there is no justification for assisted delivery. If a woman is urged to bear down whether she feels the need or not, based only on a diagnosis of full dilatation, the result is too often maternal exhaustion and instrument delivery—in settings all too familiar in clinical obstetrics when the "patience and fortitude of all have been dissipated" (124). Crawford may go too far but his perspective deserves careful review, as many clinicians are displeased with current pronouncements concerning second stage management under regional anesthesia.

Clinical experience in general supports Crawford's contentions (117, 125, 126). McQueen and coworkers studied 100 patients with epidural anesthesia dividing them into two groups. The first group was instructed to push immediately when full dilatation was diagnosed. The second group was left lying on their sides until the fetal head became visible or until progress in rotation/descent of the fetal head ceased, as judged by regular vaginal examination. In the latter group, pushing was not specifically encouraged unless the patient spontaneously initiated it. There was no reduction in the overall use of instrumental delivery between the two groups. However, there was a 50% reduction in the need for rotational deliveries primarily due to reduction in the number of occipitolateral positions. Further, in those women managed without immediate pushing, the vertex had descended on the average of 1 cm more than in the comparison group. The patients in the study were internally monitored and there were no differences in Apgar scores or mean umbilical pH at delivery. The mean length of the second stage for patients in the "no push" group was 2½ hours.

Recent changes in anesthetic epidural management by reducing the total dose of anesthetic administered and changing the method of administration will also probably result in less alteration of the second stage and a reduced need for instrumentation. Continuous infusion of an epidural agent and combining minidose bupivacaine and synthetic narcotics such as fentanyl results in almost undetectable motor blockade (108, 127–130). The effect of this management on the incidence and degree of difficulty of operative intervention is yet unclear. However, such changes combined with more liberal ideas about the acceptable length of the second stage, judicious uterine stimulation, and patient repositioning should result in fewer assisted deliveries or at least fewer midpelvic or rotational instrumental deliveries. In sum, epidural anesthesia lengthens the second stage of labor in a substantial proportion of patients. The interference of regional anesthesia in the second stage is complex but is to a good extent overcome by maternal repositioning, assistance with voluntary pushing, judicious administration of oxytocin and a willingness to permit the second stage to extend beyond arbitrary limits as long as progress is continuous and no signs of fetal or maternal distress ensue (108, 131).

REFERENCES

1. Mauriceau F. Traité des maladies des femmes grosses. Quatrieme ed. Paris: L D'Houry, 1694.
2. Pajot C. Travaux d'obstetrique et de gynécologie précédés d'élements de practique obstétricale. Paris: H Lauwereyns, 1882.
3. Laufe LE. Obstetric forceps. New York: Harper & Row, 1968.
4. Das K. Obstetric forceps: its history and evolution. Calcutta: The Art Press, 1929.
5. Kielland C. Uber die anlegung der zange am nicht rotierten kopf mit beschreibung eines neuen zangemodelles und einer neuen anlegungsmethode. Monatsschr Geburtsh Gynakol 1916; 43:38–78.
6. Martius G. Operative obstetrics. 12th ed. New York: Thieme-Stratton, 1980.
7. Dennon EH. Forceps deliveries. 2nd ed. Philadelphia: FA Davis, 1964.
8. Luikart R. A modification of the Kielland, Simpson, and Tucker-McLane forceps to simplify their use and improve function and safety. Am J Obstet Gynecol 1937; 34:686–687.
9. Luikart R. A new forceps possessing a sliding lock, modified fenestra, with improved handle and axis traction attachment. Am J Obstet Gynecol 1940; 40:1058–1060.
10. Dill LV. The obstetrical forceps. Springfield, Illinois: Charles C Thomas, 1953.
11. Parry-Jones E. Barton's forceps. Baltimore: Williams & Wilkins, 1972.
12. Barton LG, Caldwell WE, Studdiford WE. A new obstetric forceps. Am J Obstet Gynecol 1928; 15:16–22.
13. Laufe LE. A new divergent outlet forceps. Am J Obstet Gynecol 1968; 101:509–512.
14. Piper EB, Bachman C. The prevention of fetal injuries in breech delivery. JAMA 1929; 92:217–221.
15. Laufe LE. A Kielland-Barton (K-B) obstetric forceps. Obstet Gynecol 1959; 14:541–543.
16. Shute WB. An obstetrical forceps which uses a new principle of parallelism. Am J Obstet Gynecol 1959; 77:442–446.
17. Goodlin RC. Modified manual rotation in pelvic delivery. Obstet Gynecol 1986; 67:128–130.
18. Bill AH. A new axis traction handle for solid blade forceps. Am J Obstet Gynecol 1925; 9:600–607.
19. Dennon EH. A classification of forceps operations according to station of head in pelvis. Am J Obstet Gynecol 1952; 63:272–283.
20. Committee on Obstetrics: Maternal and Fetal Medicine 59: Obstetric Forceps. American College of Obstetricians and Gynecologists, Washington, DC: 1988.
21. Cohen WR. Influence of the duration of second stage labor on perinatal outcome and puerperal morbidity. Obstet Gynecol 1977; 49:266–269.
22. Bergman P, Malmström T. Natal and postnatal foetal mortality in association with vacuum extraction and forceps delivery. Gynaecologia 1962; 154:65–72.

23. Cooke WAR. Evaluation of the midforceps operation. Am J Obstet Gynecol 1967; 99:327–332.
24. Widen JA, Erez S, Steer CM. An evaluation of the vacuum extractor in a series of 201 cases. Am J Obstet Gynecol 1967; 98:24–31.
25. Leeton J, Waldron K. Post-partum reactions to instrumental delivery. Med J Aust 1971; 58:1020–1022.
26. Cardozo LD, Gibb DMF, Studd JWW, Cooper DJ. Should we abandon Kielland forceps? Br Med J 1983; 287:315–317.
27. Decker WH, Dickson WA, Heaton CE. An analysis of five hundred forty-seven midforceps operations. Am J Obstet Gynecol 1953; 65:294–303.
28. Cosgrove RA, Weaver OS. An analysis of 1,000 consecutive midforceps operations. Am J Obstet Gynecol 1957; 73:556–558.
29. Kirk RF, Krumholz BA, Callagan DA. The mid-forceps operation. Prognosis based on pelvic capacity and fetal weight. Obstet Gynecol 1960; 15:447–451.
30. Danforth DN, Ellis AH. Midforceps delivery—a vanishing art? Am J Obstet Gynecol 1963; 86:29–37.
31. Nyirjesy I, Hawks BL, Falls HC, Munsat TL, Pierce WE. A comparative clinical study of the vacuum extractor and forceps. Am J Obstet Gynecol 1964; 85:1071–1082.
32. Dunlop DL. Midforceps operations at the University of Alberta Hospital (1965–1967). Am J Obstet Gynecol 1969; 103:471–475.
33. Bowes WA, Bowes C. Current role of the midforceps operation. Clin Obstet Gynaecol 1980; 23:549–557.
34. Dierker LJ, Rosen MG, Thompson K, Lynn P. Midforceps deliveries: long-term outcome of infants. Am J Obstet Gynecol 1986; 154:764–768.
35. Nilsen ST. Boys born by forceps and vacuum extraction examined at 18 years of age. Acta Obstet Gynecol Scand 1984; 63:549–554.
36. Bergsjo P, Schmidt E, Pusch D. Difference in the reported frequencies of some obstetrical interventions in Europe. Br J Obstet Gynaecol 1983; 90:628–632.
37. Healy DL, Laufe LE. Survey of obstetric forceps training in North America in 1981. Am J Obstet Gynecol 1985; 151:54–58.
38. DeLee JB. The prophylactic forceps operation. Am J Obstet Gynecol 1920; 1:34–44.
39. Healy DL, Quinn MA, Pepperell RJ. Rotational delivery of the fetus: Kielland's forceps and two other methods compared. Br J Obstet Gynaecol 1982; 89:501–506.
40. Marin RD. A review of the use of Barton's forceps for the rotation of the fetal head from the transverse position. Aust NZ J Obstet Gynaecol 1978; 18:234–237.
41. Chiswick ML, James DK. Kielland's forceps: association with neonatal morbidity and mortality. Br Med J 1979; 1:7–9.
42. Vacca W, Grant A, Wyatt G, Chalmers I. Portsmouth operative delivery trial: a comparison vacuum extraction and forceps delivery. Br J Obstet Gynaecol 1983; 90:1107–1112.
43. Lasbrey AU, Orchard CD, Crichton D. A study of the relative events and scope for vacuum extraction as opposed to forceps delivery. S Afr J Obstet Gynaecol 1964; 2:1–3.
44. Tank ES, Davis R, Holt JF, Morley GW. Mechanisms of trauma during breech delivery. Obstet Gynecol 1971; 38:761–767.
45. Whitacre FE. Forceps management of breech and face presentations. Clin Obstet Gynecol 1965; 8:882–893.
46. Milner RDG. Neonatal mortality of breech deliveries with and without forceps to the aftercoming head. Br J Obstet Gynaecol 1975; 82:783–785.
47. Chiswick ML, Paintin DB, Vincent F. Forceps delivery and neonatal outcome/obstetric outcome. In: Beard RW, Paintin, DB, eds. Outcomes of obstetric intervention in Britain, proceedings of a scientific meeting of the Royal College of Obstetricians and Gynaecologists. 1980: 32–45.
48. de Crespigny LCH, Robinson HP. Can obstetricians prevent neonatal intraventricular haemorrhage? Aust NZ J Obstet Gynaecol 1983; 23:146–149.
49. Fairweather DVI. Obstetric management and follow-up of a very-low-

birth-weight infant. J Reprod Med 1981; 26:387–392.
50. Crawford CS. Incidence and risk factor analysis of subependymal intraventricular hemorrhage in less than 1500 gm infants born at a perinatal center. Pediatr Res 1982; 16:1231.
51. Bejar R, Curbelo V, Coen RV, Leopold G, James A, Saunders B, Borreco R, Gluck L. Incidence of intraventricular and germinal layer hemorrhage (IVH/GLH) in preterm infants born per vagina and cesarean section. Pediatr Res 1980; 14:629.
52. Volpe JJ. Neonatal intraventricular hemorrhage. N Engl J Med 1981; 304:886–891.
53. Rayburn WF, Donn SM, Kolin MG, Schork MA. Obstetric care in intraventricular hemorrhage in the low birth weight infant. Obstet Gynecol 1983; 61:408–413.
54. Benson JWT, Drayton MR, Hayward C, Murphy JF, Osborne JP, Rennie JM, Schulte JF, Speidel BD, Cooke RWI. Multicentre trial of ethamsylate for prevention of periventricular haemorrhage in very low birth weight infants. Lancet 1986; 2:1297–1300.
55. Volpe JJ. Neonatal intracranial hemorrhage. Pathophysiology, neuropathology, and clinical features. Clin Perinatol 1977; 4:77–102.
56. Szymonowicz W, Yu VYH, Bajuk B, Astbury J. Neurodevelopmental outcome of periventricular haemorrhage and leukomalacia in infants 1250 g or less at birth. Early Hum Dev 1986; 14:1–7.
57. Tejani N, Rebold B, Tuck S, Ditroia D, Sutro W, Verma U. Obstetric factors in the causation of early periventricular-intraventricular hemorrhage. Obstet Gynecol 1984; 65:510–515.
58. Szymonowicz W, Yu VYH. Timing and evolution of periventricular haemorrhage in infants weighing 1250 g or less at birth. Arch Dis Child 1984; 59:7–12.
59. Szymonowicz W, Yu VYH, Wilson FE. Antecedents of periventricular haemorrhage in infants weighing 1250 g or less at birth. Arch Dis Child 1984; 59:13–17.
60. Weindling AM, Wilkinson AR, Cook

J, Calvert SA, Fok TF, Rochefort MJ. Perinatal events which preceed periventricular haemorrhage and leukomalacia in the newborn. Br J Obstet Gynaecol 1985; 92:1218–1223.
61. D'Souza SW, Gowland M, Richards B, Cadman J, Mellor V, Sims DG, Chiswick ML. Head size, brain growth, and lateral ventricles in very low birth weight infants. Arch Dis Child 1986; 61:1090–1095.
62. Greisen G, Petersen MB, Pedersen SA, Baekgaard, P. Status at two years in 121 very low birth weight survivors related to neonatal intraventricular haemorrhage and mode of delivery. Acta Paediatr Scand 1986; 75:24–30.
63. Wigglesworth JS. Perinatal pathology. Philadelphia: WB Saunders, 1984.
64. Cooke RWI, Rolfe P, Howat P. Apparent cerebral blood-flow in newborns with respiratory disease. Dev Med Child Neurol 1979; 21:154–160.
65. Lou HC, Lassen NA, Friis S, Hansen B. Impaired autoregulation of cerebral blood flow in the distressed newborn infant. J Pediatr 1979; 94:118–121.
66. Johnson GN, Palahniuk RJ, Tweed WA, Jones MV, Wade JG. Regional cerebral blood flow changes during severe asphyxia reduced by slow partial umbilical cord compression. Am J Obstet Gynecol 1979; 135:48–52.
67. Tejani N, Verma U, Hameed C, Chayen B. Method and route of delivery in the low birth weight vertex presentation correlated with early periventricular/intraventricular hemorrhage. Obstet Gynecol 1987; 69:1–4.
68. Worthington D, Davis LE, Grausz JP, Sobocinski K. Factors influencing survival and morbidity with very low birth weight delivery. Obstet Gynecol 1983; 62:550–555.
69. Shinnar S, Molteni R, Gammon K, D'Souza BJ, Altman J, Freeman JM. Intraventricular hemorrhage in the premature infant: a changing outlook. N Engl J Med 1982; 306:1464–1468.
70. Levine MI, Fawer CL, Lamont RF.

Risk factors and the development of intraventricular hemorrhage in the preterm neonate. Arch Dis Child 1982; 57:410–417.

71. Clark CE, Clyman R, Roth R, Sniderman SH, Lane B, Ballard RA. Risk factor analysis of intraventricular hemorrhage in low-birth-weight infants. J Pediatr 1981; 99:624–628.

72. Dykes F, Lazzara A, Ahmann P, Blumenstein B, Schwartz J, Brann AW. Intraventricular hemorrhage: a prospective evaluation of etiopathogenesis. Pediatrics 1980; 66:42–49.

73. Welch RA, Bottoms SF. Reconsideration of head compression and intraventricular hemorrhage in the vertex very-low-birth-weight fetus. Obstet Gynecol 1986; 68:29–34.

74. Barrett JM, Boehm FH, Vaughn WK. The effect of type of delivery on neonatal outcome in singleton infants of birthweight of 1000 g or less. JAMA 1983; 250:625–629.

75. Haesslein H, Goodlin RC. Delivery of the tiny newborn. Am J Obstet Gynecol 1979; 134:192–200.

76. Morales WJ, Koernten J. Obstetric management and intraventricular hemorrhage in very-low-birth-weight infants. Obstet Gynecol 1986; 68:35–40.

77. Beverley DW, Chance GW, Coates CF. Intraventricular haemorrhage—timing of occurrence and relationship to perinatal events. Br J Obstet Gynaecol 1984; 91:1007–1013.

78. Hobel CJ, Oakes GK. Special considerations in the management of preterm labor. Clin Obstet Gynecol 1980; 23:147–164.

79. Huff DL, Thurnau GR, Shelton R. The outcome of protective forceps deliveries of 26–33 week infants. Abstract 45. Society of Perinatal Obstetricians Seventh Annual Meeting, Lake Buena Vista, Florida, February 5–7, 1987.

80. Bishop EH, Israel SL, Briscoe CC. Obstetric influences of the premature infant's first year of development. A report from the collaborative study of cerebral palsy. Obstet Gynecol 1965; 26:628–635.

81. Dolfin, T, Skidmore MD, Fong KW, Hoskins EN, Shennan AT. Incidence, severity and timing of subependymal and intraventricular hemorrhages in preterm infants born in a perinatal unit as detected by serial real time ultrasound. Pediatrics 1983; 71:541–546.

82. O'Driscoll K, Meager D, MacDonald D, Geoghegan F. Traumatic intracranial haemorrhage in firstborn infants and delivery with obstetric forceps. Br J Obstet Gynaecol 1981; 88:577–581.

83. Brown FJ. Failed forceps. Br Med J 1949; 97:975–976.

84. Bunn E. Grundriss zum studium der geburtshilfe. Munchen und Wiesbaden: Verlag von JF Bergmann, 1922: 576–577.

85. Dyer I. Trial and failed forceps. Clin Obstet Gynaecol 1965; 8:914–918.

86. Hobbins JC, Winsberg F, Berkowitz RL. Ultrasonography in obstetrics and gynecology. 2nd ed. Baltimore: Williams & Wilkins, 1983.

87. Hadlock FP, Harrist RB, Sharman RS, Deter RL, Park SK. Estimation of fetal weight with the use of head, body, and femur measurements—a prospective study. Am J Obstet Gynecol 1985; 151:333–337.

88. Elliott JP, Gariete TJ, Freeman RK, McQuown DS, Patel JM. Ultrasonic prediction of fetal macrosomia in diabetic patients. Obstet Gynecol 1982; 61:159–162.

89. Modanlou HD, Komatsu G, Dorchester W, Freeman RK, Bosu, SK. Large-for-gestational-age neonates: anthropometric reasons for shoulder dystocia. Obstet Gynecol 1982; 60:417–423.

90. Oxorn H. Human labor and birth. 4th ed. New York: Appleton-Century-Crofts, 1980.

91. Douglass LH, Kaltreider DF. Trial forceps. Am J Obstet Gynecol 1953; 65:889–896.

92. Boyd ME, Usher RH, McLean FH, Normal BE. Failed forceps. Obstet Gynecol 1986; 68:779–783.

93. Murray EF. Failed forceps. Clin J 1927; 56:488–492.

94. Miller D. Observations on unsuccessful forceps cases: causation, management, and end results. Br Med J 1928; 2:183–185.

95. Claye AM. Failed forceps cases. The Practit 1931; 126:611–616.

96. Freeth HD. The cause and management of failed forceps cases. Br Med J 1950; 2:18–21.

97. Law RG. Failed forceps: a review of 37 cases. Br Med J 1953; 2:955–957.

98. Hughey MJ, McElin TW, Lussky R. Forceps operations and perspective. I. Midforceps rotation operations. J Reprod Med 1978; 20:253–259.

99. Stacey JE. Failed forceps. Br Med J 1931; 2:1073–1078.

100. Taylor E. Can mid-forceps operations be eliminated? Obstet Gynecol 1953; 2:302–307.

101. Benkus MD, Ramamurthy RS, O'Connor PS, Brown K, Hayashi RH. Cohort studies of silastic obstetric vacuum cup deliveries: I. Safety of the instrument. Obstet Gynecol 1985; 66:503–509.

102. Danforth DN. Transverse arrest. Clin Obstet Gynaecol 1965; 8:854–867.

103. Niswander KR, Gordon M. Safety of the low-forceps operation. Am J Obstet Gynecol 1973; 117:619–630.

104. Schenker JG, Serr DM. Comparative study of delivery by vacuum extractor and forceps. Am J Obstet Gynecol 1967; 98:32–39.

105. Hoult IJ, MacLennan AH, Carrie LES. Lumbar epidural analgesia in labour: relation to fetal malposition and instrumental delivery. Br Med J 1977; I:14–16.

106. Johnson WL, Winter WW, Eng M, Bonica JJ, Hunter CA. Effect of pudendal, spinal, and peridural block anesthesia on the second stage of labor. Am J Obstet Gynecol 1972; 113:166–175.

107. Raabe N, Balfrage P. Lumbar epidural analgesia in labour. Acta Obstet Gynecol Scand 1976; 53:125–129.

108. Youngstrom PC. A buyer's guide to pain relief for childbirth. Cleveland: Department of Anesthesiology, Case Western Reserve University School of Medicine, 1986.

109. Maltau JM, Andersen HT. Continuous epidural anaesthesia with a low frequency of instrumental deliveries. Acta Obstet Gynecol Scand 1975; 54:401–406.

110. Jouppila R, Jouppila P, Karinen JM, Hollmen A. Segmental epidural analgesia in labour: related to the progress of labour, fetal malposition and instrumental delivery. Acta Obstet Gynecol Scand 1979; 58:135–139.

111. Bates RG, Helm CW, Duncan A, Edmonds DK. Uterine activity in the second stage of labour and the effect of epidural analgesia. Br J Obstet Gynaecol 1985; 92:1246–1250.

112. Goodfellow CF, Hull MGR, Swaab DF, Dogterom J, Buijs RM. Oxytocin deficiency at delivery with epidural analgesia. Br J Obstet Gynaecol 1983; 90:214–219.

113. Leake RD, Weitzman RE, Glatz TA, Fisher DA. Stimulation of oxytocin secretion in the human. Clin Res 1979; 27:99A.

114. Ferguson JKW. A study of the motility of the intact uterus at term. Surg Gynecol Obstet 1941; 73:359–366.

115. Fitzpatrick RJ. Blood concentration of oxytocin in labour. J Endocrinol 1961; 22:19–20.

116. Bates RG, Helm CW. Epidural analgesia during labour: why does this increase the forceps delivery rate? J R Soc Med 1985; 78:890–892.

117. Goodfellow CF, Studd C. The reduction of forceps in primagravidae with epidural analgesia—a controlled trial. Br J Clin Pract 1979; 33:287–288.

118. Thornburn J, Moir DD. Extradural analgesia: the influence of volume and concentration of bupivacaine on the mode of delivery, and analgesic efficacy and motor block. Br J Anaesth 1984; 53:933–939.

119. Doughty A. Selective epidural analgesia and the forceps rate. Br J Anaesth 1969; 41:1058–1062.

120. Potter N, MacDonald RD. Obstetric consequences of epidural analgesia in nulliparous patients. Lancet 1971; 1:1031–1034.

121. Shnider SM, Levinson G, Ralston DH. Regional anesthesia for labor and delivery. In: Shnider SM, Levinson G, eds. Anesthesia for obstetrics. Baltimore: Williams & Wilkins, 1979; 93–108.

122. Puddicombe JF. Maternal posture for correction of posterior fetal position. J Int Col Surg 1955; 23:73–77.

123. Phillips KC, Thomas TA. Second stage of labour with or without extradural analgesia. Anaesthesia 1983;

38:972–976.

124. Crawford JS. The stages and phases of labour: a worn out nomenclature that invites hazard. Lancet 1983; 2:271–272.

125. Maresh M, Choong KH, Beard RW. Delayed pushing with lumbar epidural analgesia in labour. Br J Obstet Gynaecol 1983; 90:623–627.

126. McQueen J, Mylrea L. Lumbar epidural analgesia in labour. Br Med J 1977; 1:640–641.

127. Li DF, Rees GAD, Rosen M. Continuous extradural infusion of 0.0625% or 0.125% bupivacaine for pain relief in primigravid labour. Br J Anaesth 1985; 57:264–270.

128. Desprats R. Use of fentanyl and marcaine as compared with marcaine alone in epidural analgesia. J Gynecol Obstet Biol Reprod 1983; 12:901–905.

129. Van Steenberg A. The best of two worlds: combination of local anesthetic and narcotic for epidural analgesia during labor. Obstet Anesth Dig 1983; 3:65–67.

130. Youngstrom PC, Eastwood D, Patel H, Bhatia R, Cowan R, Sutheimer C. Epidural fentanyl and bupivacaine and labor: double-blind study. Anesthesiology 1984; 61:414.

131. Bailey PW, Howard FA. Epidural analgesia and forceps delivery: laying a bogey. Anaesthesia 1983; 38:282–285.

3

Forceps Operations

Students should never think themselves perfect; for after all the instruction that can possibly be conveyed, there are many things in midwifery than can only be learned by practice and observation; and cases will sometimes arise which will puzzle and foil the best practitioner.

WILLIAM SMELLIE, 1774 (1)

. . . Pour tirer, suivant l'axe classique d'une façon mathematique . . . Je resume: canal immobile, centre immuable, instruments inflexibles . . . Tracer pour l'introduction et l'extraction le cercle dont instrument est une partie . . .

CHARLES PAJOT, 1882 (2)

Outlet Forceps Application: Discussion

Outlet forceps is the principal instrumental obstetric forceps operation. The basic features of this application are common to all instrumental deliveries. These include correct maternal positioning, adequate anesthesia, an empty bladder, operator certainty of fetal position and station, operator knowledge of how to proceed, and a firm indication for instrumentation. Several aspects of the technique of application deserve comment. Dorsal lithotomy position is classically preferred for forceps application but is not required in all instances as long as patient and operator are comfortable. The patient's bladder should be empty to avoid injury, particularly if rotation or delivery from occiput posterior is contemplated. Voluntary voiding or the Credé maneuver is often sufficient. Straight catheterization should be used without hesitation if voluntary emptying is impossible or if a rotational or midpelvic procedure is contemplated. In general, epidural or saddle block anesthesia is preferred. With proper coaching and a cooperative patient, pudendal block is often adequate for outlet procedures. Except in the most unusual circumstances, general anesthesia is unnecessary and should be avoided due to maternal and fetal risks.

Traction is timed to contractions. If the patient is not aware of her contractions, an attendant should palpate the uterus to inform the operator when uterine tension builds. Tension on the blades should mirror the contraction—a slow build to a full pressure with subsequent relaxation in force as the uterine contraction abates. Rapid traction without accompanying contractions or jerking of the blades is unlikely to achieve delivery and risks maternal/fetal injury. The force for delivery is provided by the operator's right arm, with the elbow bent at a right angle. Some operators place a folded towel between the articulated blade handles to reduce lateral compression of the fetal head. The left hand rests on the shank of the blades and presses downward (Saxtorph-Pajot or Osiander maneuver) (Fig. 3.10). This creates a vector of force guiding the fetal head through the pelvic curve (Carus' curve) (Figs. 3.1 and 3.2). The angle of pull is modified either toward the symphysis or, alternatively, in the direction of the perineum as resistance is felt and the presenting part descends. The blades should not be rocked up and down during the delivery as the posterior toe of the blade will injure the posterior vaginal vault as descent of the fetal head occurs. The fetal heart should be auscultated or checked by real

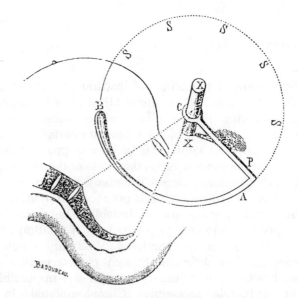

Figure 3.1.   The pelvic curve or Carus' curve as illustrated by Pajot (1882) (2). Note that the forceps traverse a portion (B through A) of an imaginary circle (center at X) that passes through the center of the bony pelvis (see also Fig. 3.2). (Courtesy of the Historical Division/Cleveland Health Sciences Library, Cleveland, OH.)

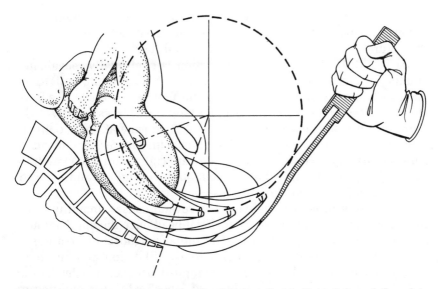

Figure 3.2. Note the course of the fetal head (B through A in Fig. 3.1) through the pelvic curve (Carus' curve) during a forceps operation.

time ultrasound, a hand-held doppler device, scalp electrode recording, or direct auscultation between contractions/pulls. The blades may be disarticulated between contractions at the operator's discretion.

As traction is applied and descent occurs, an episiotomy may be cut, if necessary. The episiotomy is best performed when the perineum is under tension. Such timing has two advantages: blood loss is reduced by compression and a better judgment can be made of the extent of the incision required.

The appropriate application of force is a serious issue in the use of forceps. Excessive force is a risk to mother and infant. The primary function of obstetric forceps is to provide traction. It is likely the greatest fetal risk for intracranial injury from forceps results from compression of the fetal head by the forceps blades, and for classic instruments, cranial compression is proportionate to the amount of traction applied. Several simple precautions should always be taken to control the force and direction of traction. Traction should be applied by an operator who is seated. Periods of relaxation, either corresponding to spontaneous contractions or imposed by the rhythm of the operator, are important between pulls. Traction should never be greater than that which can be accomplished by the operator's flexing his/her forearm. He/she should not brace his/her feet and the force exerted should never be great enough to move the patient's hips from the table's edge. While a firm pull is at times required, the average surgeon is easily capable of successfully delivering an infant with forceps without ever taxing his/her strength. Forceps are designed to be a guide to the natural descent and delivery of the fetal head rather than a force extractor (3). In theory, as long as station is continually reevaluated and the fetal heart tones are acceptable, there is no absolute limit to the period of forceps application nor to the number of traction efforts. However, the incidence of trauma and failure increases rapidly if the number of tractions exceeds five (Table 4.3). In general, then, delivery should be accomplished within five pulls, *with progress commencing with the first pull.* However, if no descent occurs with adequate traction and a correctly applied instrument on the *initial* attempt, the procedure must be immediately reassessed.

Failure in forceps delivery has several causes. Inability to either insert the blades or advance the fetal head once the application is complete may occur (Table 3.1). The initial diagnosis of position or fetal station may be incorrect. Full cervical dilatation may not have been reached and/or the cervix is entrapped between the fetal head and the forceps blade. With prolonged labor, extensive molding or caput succedaneum formation may have obscured cranial landmarks, confusing the operator, or resulted in an oblique or asynclitic position. In unusual cases, advancement is prevented by fetal/maternal tumors, collision of twins, or through formation of a pathologic retraction ring (Bandl's ring) or a constriction ring. The fetal head may also be deflexed. Finally, true cephalopelvic disproportion may exist.

If traction fails to advance the fetal head and on careful reassessment the forceps application is *correct*, then the attempt at vaginal delivery should be abandoned and cesarean section performed (see Chapter 2, "Trial versus Failed Forceps").

If traction fails to advance the fetal head and the initial attempt at an application is determined to have been *incorrect*, then reapplication or use of the vacuum extractor is considered. Careful palpation of the fontanelles and suture lines, feeling for the fetal orbits, "flipping" the fetal ear, real time ultrasound examination, and Leopold's maneuvers are all helpful in the correct determination of position/station. In all of these diagnostic examinations, care must be taken to avoid dis-

Table 3.1. Events Requiring Immediate Reassessment of an Attempted Instrumental Delivery

Operator cannot be certain of fetal position or station
The cervix is found to be incompletely dilated
Inadequate anesthesia is present
Operator cannot articulate or lock the forceps
Operator cannot insert or successfully wander a blade
Fetal head is dislodged to higher station during attempted forceps introduction

lodging the fetal head. Instrumental vaginal delivery is no place for uncertainty or heroics. If the operator is uncertain of position or application, the contemplated procedure *must* be abandoned.

The correct *cephalic* application of the forceps is termed the biparietal or bimalar application (Fig. 3.3) (4, 5). Properly applied in this fashion, the compressive force generated by the blades is evenly distributed over the fetal head. In a *pelvic* application, the forceps are applied independently of the exact orientation of the fetal head. The only currently acceptable pelvic application is forceps to the aftercoming head in breech presentation (5). When the blades are correctly applied, the plane of the blades corresponds to the occipitomental diameter of the fetal head. The tips of the forceps blades lie over the fetal cheeks with the upper or concave border of the blade directed either toward the fetal occiput in anterior positions or the face in posterior positions. The biparietal diameter of the fetal head fits in the center of the cephalic curve of the instrument. In establishing the correct application, the fenestration of the blades, the location of the posterior fontanelle, and the sagittal suture are the important landmarks (the "three checks") (Fig. 3.9). The sagittal suture should lie in the midline. If the suture curves to one side, it indicates an oblique application (Fig. 3.4). If the blades are applied obliquely, their grasp will be insecure and the fetal head will be exposed to unusual pressure (Fig. 3.4). The posterior fontanelle is one finger breadth anterior to the plane of the shanks and an equal distance from the side of the blades. When the blades are

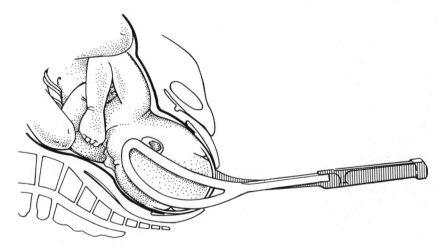

Figure 3.3.   Correct biparietal, bimalar, cephalic forceps application (see text for details). (Redrawn from Dennon EH. Forceps deliveries. 2nd ed. Philadelphia: FA Davis, 1964: 35.)

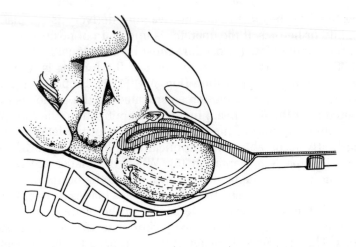

Figure 3.4 Incorrect oblique (brow-mastoid) forceps application. Note how anterior blade of the Kielland forceps overlies the fetal face. Such applications predispose to injury of the fetal eye or scalp (Redrawn from Pritchard JA, MacDonald PC, Gant NF. Williams obstetrics. 17th ed. New York: Appleton-Century-Crofts, 1985.)

correctly applied, only one fingertip can be inserted between the fenestration of the blade and the fetal head. If too much of the fenestration is palpable, the blade is not correctly inserted or the head is very small. If one blade is misapplied over the brow and the other over the occiput, the instrument cannot be locked or articulated or, if locked, the blades will slip off when traction is applied (Fig. 3.5). Correctly applied, the forceps will fit easily and will not slip with normal traction.

On molded heads of term-size infants, the best application is obtained with blades which have a long, tapering cephalic curve such as the Simpson. Forceps with a short, full curve (Elliot type) do not fit evenly in this setting, causing points of unusual pressure (4, 5). Further, short blades may not be anchored below the malar eminences, risking laceration or slippage. The position of the blades along the sagittal suture is most important. The center of the biparietal diameter of the head, what Dennon describes as the *pivot point* of the fetal cranium, should lie in the middle of a imaginary line connecting the widest diameter of the cephalic curve of the blades and the plane of the shanks (4). If the pivot point of the head is not in the center of the blades, the head will be overextended or excessively flexed with traction.

The application outlined here is that suggested by Dennon (4) and Laufe (5). However, based on the study of tension to the falx cerebri and the tentorium cerebelli, Mines (3) believes that the plane of

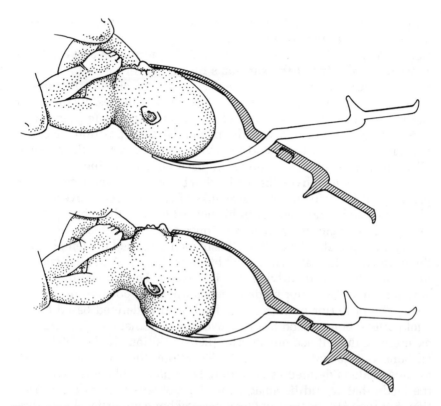

Figure 3.5. Incorrect occipitofrontal Kielland forceps application. When so applied the forceps cannot lock or will not articulate correctly. With traction, cranial extension or blade slippage is likely, risking fetal and maternal injury (Redrawn from Pritchard JA, MacDonald PC, Gant NF. Williams Obstetrics. 17th ed. New York: Appleton-Century-Crofts, 1985.)

the shanks should be positioned *directly over the posterior fontanelle.* This is a centimeter or two from the position suggested by Dennon (4). Based on studies of preserved specimens, Mines argues that distortion and tension on the falx cerebri and tentorium cerebelli are minimal with the blades in this position. The author was trained to follow the Dennon/Laufe technique and, due to its proven clinical utility, recommends its use.

In the following sections, the application of forceps is illustrated in a series of steps corresponding to the principal manipulations necessary for each procedure. Adjacent to each illustration is inscribed a *circle* symbolically depicting the fontanelles of the fetal skull against horizontal/vertical axes. The orientation is, as viewed by the operator, from the plane of the midperineum with the patient in dorsal lithotomy position. In general, classic forceps are depicted unless a special application (e.g., forceps to the aftercoming head in breech presentation) is presented. The choice of forceps type for outlet and rotational procedures remains at the surgeon's discretion. In the author's opinion, operators should be experienced with the classic instruments before attempting to apply any of the specialized blades. As discussed in the text, the specific anatomy of the maternal pelvis (e.g., gynecoid versus platypelloid), parity of the patient, station, position, size, and molding of the fetal head, and the clinical experience of the surgeon, all influence the choice of forceps in each clinical setting.

For the neophyte, the distinction between *left* and *right* forceps blade appears confusing. As the shanks of classic forceps overlap, the blade grasped by the operator in his/her *left* hand is that applied to the *left* side of the maternal pelvis. Also, once applied this blade lies along the *left* fetal parietal bone. Thus, this branch is termed the *left* blade. In the following illustrations, the *left* blade is *shaded*. A similar convention is applied for identifying the *right* blade. The convention for the anterior versus posterior blade depends upon the position of the fetal head. The *posterior* portion of the fetal head is defined based on the fetal parietal bone which presents over the maternal coccyx. Thus, for example, in the left occiput anterior (LOA) position, the *left* fetal parietal bone is adjacent to the coccyx. Therefore, the corresponding *left* forceps blade is defined as *posterior*. The *anterior* blade is defined as the blade that would be adjacent to the mother's urethra after insertion. For the LOA, as the *right* fetal parietal bone underlies the urethra, this would be the *right* blade.

Outlet Forceps Applications (American College of Obstetricians and Gynecologists (ACOG) 1988 (Table 2.1)

Definition

The application of forceps when:

(a) The scalp is visible at the introitus without spreading the labia;
(b) The fetal skull has reached the pelvic floor;
(c) The sagittal suture is in the anterior/posterior diameter or in the right or left occiput anterior or posterior position;
(d) The fetal head is at or on the perineum.

Prerequisites

(a) An appropriate clinical indication;
(b) Acceptable analgesia
  ● Pudendal block,
  ● Low spinal (saddle) block,
  ● Epidural anesthesia,
  ● (Rarely) inhalation or general anesthesia;
(c) Operator certainty of fetal position following a pelvic examination to establish the station, position, and deflection of fetal head;
(d) Empty bladder (Credé, or catheterization, or recent void);
(e) Full cervical dilatation;
(f) Ruptured membranes.

Forceps Operations

Outlet Forceps to the Occiput Anterior Positions

1. Prior to forceps application the operator checks the fetal position by vaginal examination and verifies that adequate anesthesia is present, the patient is fully dilated, and the membranes are ruptured.

2. The blades are then *ghosted* prior to attempting insertion (Fig. 3.6). In ghosting (external orientation), the operator holds the forceps in front of the perineum *in the angle and position of their final application* and mentally reviews the technique of application. This step is important and is to be performed in all instrumental deliveries *prior to insertion of any forceps.* It is an additional check on fetal position, establishes the correct orientation of the instrument, and forces the operator to reconsider his/her intentions (4, 5, 7, 8).

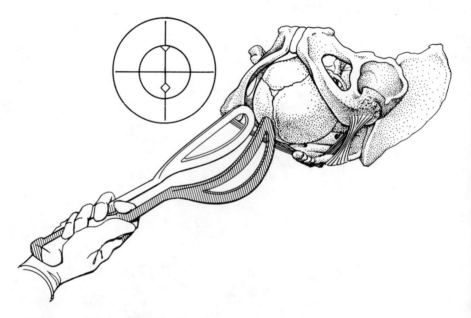

Figure 3.6.   OA position. Ghosting of Simpson forceps.

3. The *left (shaded) or posterior blade is selected first* and lubricated with surgical soap or examination gel. The handle of the blade is held lightly in the operator's left hand. Between uterine contractions, the surgeon's right hand passes into the vagina, the fingers creating a potential space between the fetal head and the vaginal side wall (Fig. 3.7). The instrument is gently introduced through the vaginal introitus and posterolaterally along the fetal parietal bone. The left hand simply guides the handle gently and does not apply force. The right hand walks the blade between the fetal head and the pelvic side wall with firm but gentle finger pressure, displacing the maternal soft tissue to permit the blade to advance over the fetal scalp in the potential space created. The operator's first two fingers lie along the leading edge of the blade, with his/her thumb on the shank. The handle of the blade is swept gently down and to the right as it passes into the pelvis. *When properly inserted, the blade advances almost by its own weight with minimal force and without obstruction.*

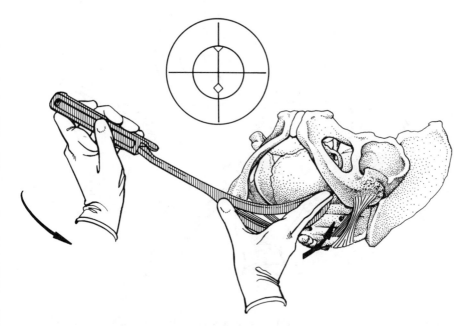

Figure 3.7.   OA position. Application of left forceps blade.

4. Once introduced the position of the blade is readjusted as necessary. The handle is held loosely and the shank of the blade manipulated by finger pressure of the vaginal hand. It is to be emphasized that to avoid fetal/maternal injury only the vaginal hand is used to move the blade.

5. Following application and initial adjustment of the left blade, the right blade is lubricated and inserted (Fig. 3.8). The left blade is supported by an assistant, if required. The right hand lightly guides the handle of the forceps. The right-sided blade is introduced *above* the plane of the previously inserted left blade so the lock can be articulated without reversal or rotation of the handles. In a simple reverse of the previous insertion technique, the operator's *left* hand passes into the vagina along the maternal right hand side of the vault. The surgeon now guides the right blade into the pelvis using his/her left thumb and first two fingers.

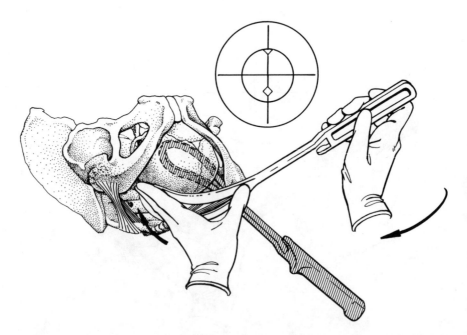

Figure 3.8.   OA position. The right forceps blade is inserted. Articulation of the blades follows.

6. After the right blade has been inserted, the forceps are articulated and the accuracy of the application checked prior to attempted traction. The blades should not require more than minimal force to either apply or articulate. If obstruction is encountered, the insertion is arrested and the application carefully reconsidered. At the operator's discretion a towel can be folded and placed between the handles to reduce compression on the fetal head after the blades are articulated.

7. The application is now complete and is checked for accuracy (3–5, 7, 8) (Fig. 3.9). It is observed that:

(a) The sagittal suture lies in the midline of the shanks;
(b) The operator is unable to place more than a fingertip between the fenestration of the blades and the fetal head on either side;
(c) The posterior fontanelle of the fetal head is no more than one finger breadth above the plane of the shanks of the forceps.

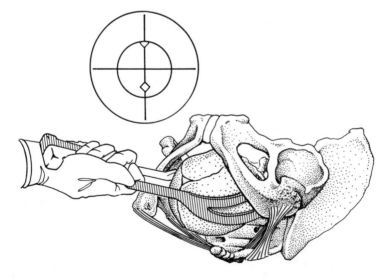

Figure 3.9. OA position. The application is checked for accuracy prior to traction (the three checks).

If the application is *incorrect*, the blades are disarticulated. They are then readjusted by use of finger pressure along the lower curve of the blade. Tension or force to the handles or shanks is *not* used to move or wander either blade (see "Wandering"). Cranial deflection is corrected prior to any attempt at traction.

8. Immediately *prior* to traction the operator performs the following:

(a) Checks for correct application
   - Position of the sagittal suture,
   - Finger insertion at blade fenestration,
   - Position of the posterior fontanelle;
(b) Checks fetal heart rate/rhythm;
(c) Checks by pelvic examination to assure that nothing lies between the fetal head and the forceps (e.g., umbilical cord, cervix, membranes);
(d) Checks for adequate anesthesia and correct maternal positioning;
(e) Checks to be certain that bladder distention is not present;
(f) Checks for cranial deflection (see Fig. 3.22);
(g) Checks mentally, rethinking the maneuvers necessary for the contemplated operation.

9. Traction is applied by the two-handed Saxtorph-Pajot maneuver (Fig. 3.10). The operator is seated with one hand pulling horizontally while the second adds downward force over the lock. This assures that the traction force vector follows the natural pelvic curve (Carus' curve) as descent occurs (see Figs. 3.1 and 3.2). The operator applies force with uterine contractions. The aim of assisted delivery is to *augment and not necessarily replace* the normal forces of delivery. Therefore, the force is built up progressively and slowly released, paralleling the pattern of the contraction, and abrupt or jerking movements are avoided. Advancement of the fetal head must occur with the *first* and each subsequent traction effort. If advancement is not made, the forceps application and the procedure must be immediately reconsidered (see Chapter 2, "Trial versus Failed Forceps").

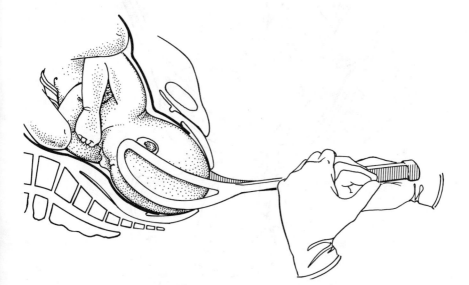

Figure 3.10.   OA position. Saxtorph-Pajot (Osiander's) maneuver.

10. As the fetal head crowns, an episiotomy is performed, if needed. Ritgen's maneuver, modified, secures the fetal chin and the mother is instructed not to push (Fig. 3.11). The head is delivered slowly and smoothly. The forceps handles are swung upward with the head as it crowns. The forceps are best left applied and used to control expulsion until the entire head has delivered, at which time removal is easy. Alternatively, once the fetal head is crowning, the blades can be removed in the *reverse* order of application while the surgeon's hand secures the fetal chin, preventing cranial retraction. Restitution of the fetal head and delivery of the infant's thorax and abdomen follow.

11. Following delivery of the placenta, the birth canal (cervix, vaginal vault, and perineum) is carefully examined to exclude lacerations or hematomas. The episiotomy, if performed, is repaired. Finally, the rectum is digitally examined, completing the operation.

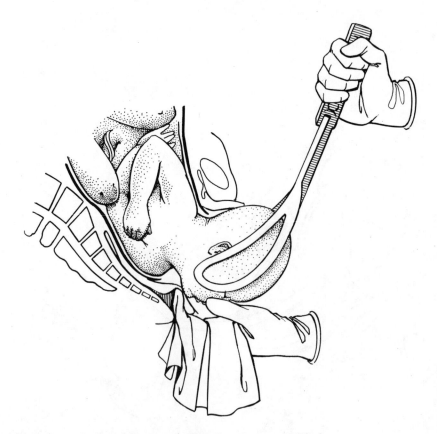

Figure 3.11.   Forceps delivery with Ritgen's maneuver, modified.

Forceps Operations with Rotation of 45° or Less

Low or Outlet Forceps to the Left Occiput Anterior (LOA) Position

If the fetal head has reached the pelvic floor with the scalp visible at the introitus, these procedures are *outlet forceps operations.* If the head is at station + 2 or more but the requirements for outlet forceps are not met, then the procedure is coded as a *low forceps operation* (see Table 2.1)

When the fetal head lies in an obliquity to the plane of the pelvis, the posterior blade is always applied first. In the LOA position, the *left* parietal bone is *posterior* and the *left* forceps blade is introduced first.

Prerequisites

(a) An appropriate clinical indication;

(b) Acceptable analgesia
- Pudendal block,
- Low spinal (saddle) block,
- Epidural anesthesia,
- (Rarely) inhalation or general anesthesia;

(c) Operator certainty of fetal position following a pelvic examination to establish the station, position, and deflection of fetal head;

(d) Empty bladder (Credé or catheterization);

(e) Full cervical dilatation;

(f) Ruptured membranes.

Application

1. All the prerequisites for forceps application have been met; adequate anesthesia and an empty bladder are present. The blades are ghosted against the perineum as previously discussed. The operator then inserts the posterior (*left*) blade for the LOA position (Fig. 3.12). The blade is initally applied as to an occiput anterior (OA) position and then wandered or adjusted to the correct location against the left fetal parietal bone (see Fig. 3.21).

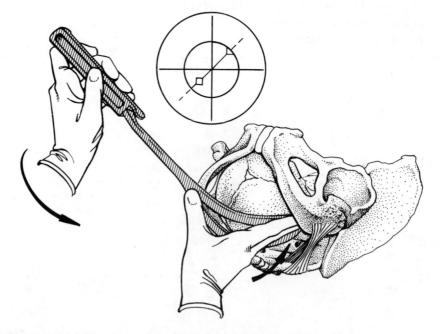

Figure 3.12.   LOA position. Introduction of left (posterior) forceps blade.

2. The *right* or *anterior* blade is now introduced (Fig. 3.13). Again, the blade is initially inserted posterolaterally as for an OA application. Once the blade is fully within the vagina the operator wanders it using digital pressure with the vaginal hand until it arrives at the correct position adjacent to the right fetal parietal bone. The blades are articulated and readjusted as necessary for a correct application using the standard checks (Fig. 3.9).

3. When the application is complete, if necessary, the fetal head is flexed by a posterior motion of the blades (see Fig. 3.22). The application is then rechecked and further adjustments made as necessary.

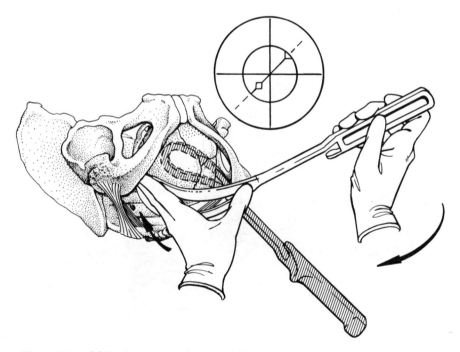

Figure 3.13. LOA position. Introduction of right (anterior) forceps blade.

4. The fetal head is then gently rotated to OA by twisting the handles of the forceps counterclockwise, taking care to maintain a constant angle between the plane of the shanks and the perineum (Fig. 3.14, see also Fig. 3.26). Rotation should be easy, requiring minimal pressure, and must not be forced. Traction with contractions follows, as with the standard OA application. Occasionally, extraction in a slight obliquity proves easier than in the direct OA position.

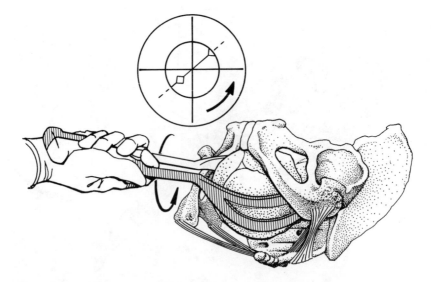

Figure 3.14.   LOA position. Simpson forceps. Rotation LOA to OA.

Low or Outlet Forceps to the Right Occiput Anterior (ROA) Position

1. For this application and in this attitude of the fetal head, the *right* fetal parietal bone is posterior. Thus the *right* forceps blade is applied first. The blade is inserted posterolaterally in the usual fashion. Once in contact with the fetal head and fully inserted, the blade is wandered until it reaches the proper position against the right fetal parietal bone (Fig. 3.15).

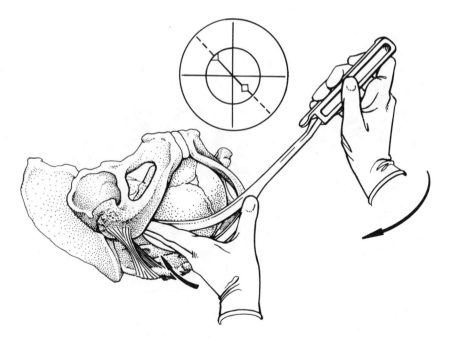

Figure 3.15. ROA position. Introduction of right (posterior) forceps blade.

2. The anterior or *left* blade is now introduced posterolaterally, using care to introduce the shanks *above* that of the previously applied blade. Once in place, the left blade is wandered anteriorly until it reaches the correct position against the left fetal parietal bone (Fig. 3.16).

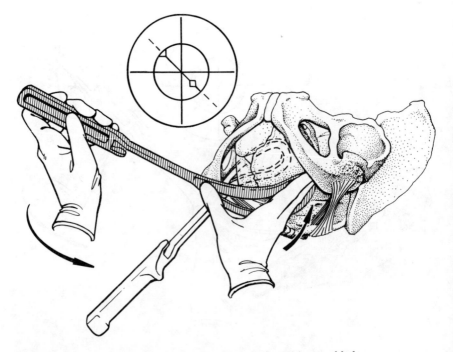

Figure 3.16.   ROA position. Introduction of left (anterior) forceps blade.

3. The blades are now articulated by gently rotating the handle of one over the other. The lock is engaged. The application is then checked (Fig. 3.9). Any necessary corrections in cranial flection are made *prior* to rotation. Rotation to OA is followed by traction with the Saxtorph-Pajot maneuver (Figs. 3.17 and 3.26). The rotational motion is smooth and should be easy. Care is taken to sweep the handles through the correct plane as governed by the angle between blades and shanks.

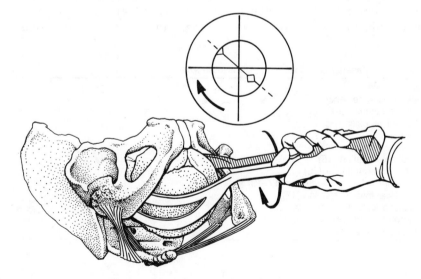

Figure 3.17.   ROA position. Simpson forceps. Rotation ROA to OA.

Low Forceps Operations with Rotation More than 45° and Midforceps Operations

If the fetal head is at station + 2 or greater and the proposed rotation is more than 45°, this procedure is considered a *low forceps operation with rotation beyond 45°*. When the fetal head is engaged but the criteria for low forceps are not met, then the procedure is coded as a *midforceps operation* (Table 2.1).

The potential hazards of rotational deliveries are well-known and include dangers of both maternal (9, 10) and fetal trauma (11, 12). A number of potential plans of management for deep transverse arrest exist (Table 3.2), including both operative and nonoperative techniques. As always, watchful expectancy and oxytocin stimulation can correct a difficult midpelvic procedure to a much easier operation if the clinical circumstances permit delay and observation (13). If this is not possible, then vacuum extraction or the application of forceps should be considered.

Transverse arrests occur during labor due either to relative cephalopelvic disproportion or to failure of the powers (14). In general, platypelloid or android pelves predispose to transverse arrest. The fetal head can also be found at transverse during rotations from an originally posterior position or from a delayed rotation commencing from the transverse. In the classic platypelloid or flat pelvis, the fetal head engages in the transverse position and descends through the midpelvis transversely due to the anteroposterior narrowing. Spontaneous rotation occurs only at the outlet in extreme cases (14). Android pelves also predispose to transverse arrest. Engagement occurs in the trans-

Table 3.2. Management Options for Transverse Arrest

Nonoperative
  Watchful expectancy
  Pitocin stimulation
  Patient repositioning
Operative
  Manual rotation
    Simple rotation (15)
    Holland maneuver (16)
    Pomeroy-Lackie maneuver (17–19)
  Classical forceps rotation (17)
  Kielland forceps rotation (20–22)
  Barton forceps rotation (10, 23)
  Vacuum extraction (24, 25)

verse diameter. With descent, cranial rotation to traverse the narrow interspinous pelvic diameter is blocked by the forward sacrum and transverse arrest occurs (14).

Operative management consists of evaluating the pelvis and the station and orientation of the fetal head in deciding which instruments to use. For example, in the uncommon markedly platypelloid pelvis, the Barton forceps are ideal (10, 26, 27). However, if this instrument is chosen, particular care must be taken, especially with rotational movements, due to the wide angulation between blades and handle (see Figs. 3.25–3.27). This is one instance where the axis traction handle is appropriate for use. Once the blades of the Barton forceps are correctly applied, traction is made to draw the fetal head down in the transverse position until rotation to occiput anterior is possible (10, 14). An Elliot-type forceps, or the Simpson or Kielland instruments, can also be applied in this clinical setting. The continued use of Kielland forceps is controversial (12, 28–31). (Kielland forceps application will be discussed at length in a later section.)

Despite observation and the use of oxytocin, the fetal head will at times remain arrested transversely in the midpelvis. If the head is unengaged, cesarean section is indicated. If not, instrumental delivery either by vacuum extraction or a forceps operation deserves consideration. It is to be remembered that cesarean section is not without risks, especially when performed emergently at the termination of a prolonged labor (31, 32). The majority of midpelvic forceps rotations are easy and achieved with minimal maternal and fetal risk. However, the operator must carefully assess pelvic capacity, the position of the fetal head, and the limits of his/her own skill prior to any attempted application. Any cranial deflection or asynclitism is corrected prior to either rotation or traction.

In a reversal of the rule learned for forceps applications to oblique positions, in transverse positions it is the *anterior forceps blade*, abutting the bladder/urethra, that is introduced first. This is for two reasons. First, if an application proves difficult it is usually the anterior blade that is the most troublesome. Thus it may be best to attempt the most difficult part of the procedure first. The second reason relates to the first. Application of the posterior blade occupies *some* pelvic space. The posterior introduction is usually easier, but can occur at the cost of station and possibly compromise the more difficult anterior blade application. Therefore, it is best to attempt the posterior blade last. This approach is not a rigid rule but a clinically

Table 3.3. Techniques for Manual Rotation

Digital splinting maneuver (33, 15)
Manual rotation maneuver (Holland maneuver) (16)
Pomeroy-Lackie maneuver (17–19)

tested technique found helpful in successful forceps application (4, 5).

Special care is required in evaluation of fetal station in transverse presentations. Anterior cranial asynclitism is common. Particular attention needs to be given to filling of the hollow of the sacrum or posterior pelvis in the accurate estimation of station. Descent of the anterior parietal bone can be substantial and fool the accoucheur on pelvic examination into the erroneous belief that the fetal head has reached a low station. Only on careful posterior palpation is it appreciated that the fetal head is not filling the pelvis and is at high station.

Manual Rotation

Prior to attempting an instrumental rotation, manual cranial rotation should be attempted. Success with the various maneuvers varies, depending upon the skill of the operator and the unique features of the individual case (Table 3.3). *Digital splinting* is the simplest maneuver. The operator inserts two fingers alongside the posterior parietal bone when the fetal head is in an oblique to transverse presentation or either parietal bone is in the occiput posterior position. With a contraction, pressure is exerted against the lambdoid suture/parietal bone to rotate the head into an occiput anterior or anterior oblique position. Occasionally, fundal pressure can assist in fixing the fetal head in the new position if the rotation is successful. Frequently, as the operator's hand is removed, the fetal head promptly returns to its original position. Thus, if rotation is successful, the head should be splinted in place by the rotating hand and the corresponding forceps blade (left or right) promptly introduced.

More extensive techniques for rotation are described but these are more likely to be associated with complications than finger rotation (15–19). In the *full manual rotation* technique, the operator's thumb and fingers are placed over the opposite parietal bones with the occiput cupped in the palm of the hand. The head is then rotated to anterior. The *Holland maneuver* is a modification of manual rotation in which the palm or surface of the operator's hand is placed over the fetal face/forehead for rotation. The fetal body is simultaneously rotated by abdominal manipulation (33). These techniques and the more extensive *Pomeroy-Lackie maneuver*, where the fetal thorax is grasped and the entire body rotated, almost invariably lose station and risk cord prolapse (Table 3.4). Further, these more extensive procedures

Table 3.4. Potential Difficulties of Manual Rotation

Loss of station
Cord prolapse
Need for anesthesia, analgesia
Failure, cranial rerotation to original position

cannot be tolerated without anesthesia. Digital rotation is appropriate to attempt and may hasten rotation or help correct a transverse midpelvic procedure into a less difficult occiput anterior or oblique application. The other procedures are uncommonly indicated except for the experienced accoucheur (4, 34).

Low Forceps Operations with Rotation More Than 45° and Midforceps Operations

Definition

This operation is the application of forceps at station +2 or more with the intention to rotate more than 45° (low forceps with rotation) or forceps application when the fetal head is engaged but the leading point of the skull is above station +2 (midforceps operation).

Prerequisites

(*a*) Appropriate application and indication;
(*b*) Acceptable analgesia
  • Pudendal nerve block,
  • Low spinal (saddle) block,
  • Epidural anesthesia,
  • (Rarely) inhalation or general anesthesia;
(*c*) Operator certainty of fetal position following a pelvic examination to establish the station, position, and deflection of the fetal head;
(*d*) Empty bladder (Credé, or catheterization);
(*e*) Full cervical dilatation;
(*f*) Ruptured membranes.

Low Forceps Rotational Procedures: Application of Classic Forceps to Right Occiput Transverse (ROT)

In this demonstration, the author has chosen to depict rotation using Simpson forceps. This choice of instrument is purely arbitrary. Solid-bladed or fenestrated Elliot-design forceps (classic Elliot or Tucker-McLane) may be applied at the operator's discretion. The basic technique of application is the same in each instance.

Application

1. To apply forceps to an occiput transverse position the operator inserts the *anterior* blade first. For midpelvic applications it is important that the bladder be empty and that adequate analgesia is present. In the ROT position, the *anterior* or *left blade* is introduced first (Fig. 3.18). The blade is inserted posterolaterally, as for a standard OA presentation, and then wandered across the fetal face to reach its final position against the left fetal parietal bone (see "Wandering," Fig. 3.21). Particular care is given to the use of firm but gentle pressure during insertion of this blade both to avoid maternal/fetal trauma as well as to avoid loss of station.

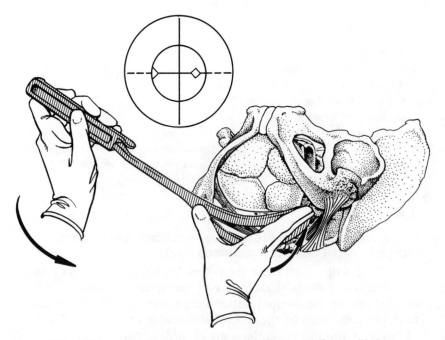

Figure 3.18. LOT position. Insertion of anterior (left) Simpson forceps blade.

2. Once the anterior blade has reached the correct position, the operator introduces the *right* or posterior blade (Fig. 3.19). This blade is introduced into the vagina in the same fashion as for an OA application. The operator's left hand enters the vagina and the left thumb and forefinger introduce the blade against the right fetal parietal bone. An assistant maintains the position of the anterior blade. In the insertion of the posterior blade, it is often helpful for the operator to guide the toe of the blade carefully along the maternal sacrum with gentle but firm digital pressure. Note that the operator crosses the blades at the time of introduction so that no rotation of the shanks is necessary for final articulation of the lock. Once the application is completed, deflection of the fetal head is corrected, if necessary. The application is then checked in the usual manner prior to rotation (Fig. 3.9).

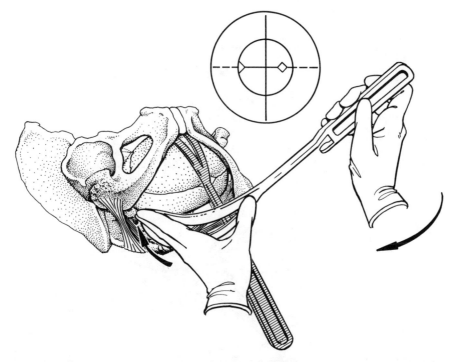

Figure 3.19. ROT position. Insertion of posterior (right) Simpson forceps blade to deflexed fetal head.

3. Following correction of deflection rotation to OA follows (Fig. 3.20). Especially with rotations of ≥90°, the operator must be certain to make smooth, gentle efforts, maintaining the correct angle of forceps application between blades and shanks to minimize the risks of maternal/fetal injury (see Figs. 3.25–3.27).

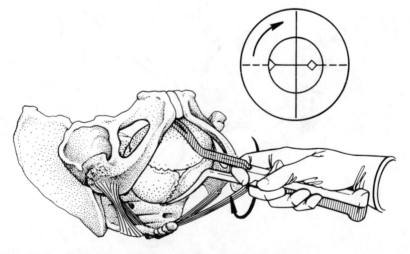

Figure 3.20.   ROT position. Simpson forceps. Rotation to OA. After correction of deflection (see Fig. 3.22).

Special Considerations

Wandering

1. In order to achieve a correct application, either the anterior or posterior blade of the forceps will often require repositioning along the fetal head. This technique is termed *wandering*. In wandering, the operator's vaginal hand is used to advance the forceps blade along or over the fetal cranium. The correct technique is to angle the edge of the blade slightly *downward* against the fetal head (Fig. 3.21). Angling the blade edge outward impedes the progress of the instrument by driving the edge of the blade into the soft tissue of the vaginal wall. The blade should never be forced, nor should it be moved by pressure exerted on the handle. The principal force is provided by the operator's vaginal fingers pressing along the edge or shank of the blade. Wandering is performed when the uterus is not contracting and only after an anesthetic has been given.

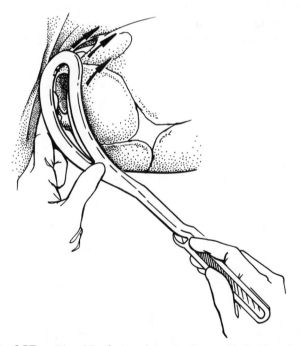

Figure 3.21. LOT position. Wandering of anterior forceps blade. Force is applied with the index finger of the operator's vaginal hand to advance the blade. The thumb maintains the blade position, guarding against slippage.

2. The essence of wandering is to traverse the fetal head with the forceps blade without undesired rotation, dislodging the fetal head, and/or loss of station. In general, solid-bladed forceps with or without Luikart's modification are best for wandering, but any blade can be used. It is best that the wandered blade be passed over the fetal face. The operator should have no consternation about this choice. Wandering across the fetal face is usually easier and less traumatic than attempting to pass the forceps blade over the occiput. The face is smaller than the occiput. Injuries to facial structures are virtually non-existent as long as excessive force is not used. A possible disadvantage of facial wandering is posterior cranial rotation, especially if the head has been dislodged during the introduction of the forceps blade. If facial wandering fails, an attempt is made around the occiput. A possible advantage of occipital wandering is that inadvertent cranial displacement assists the anterior rotation of the occiput, albeit almost certainly with loss of station. However, the large bulk of the occiput also means an increased risk of maternal vaginal lacerations and, in general, an increased likelihood of failure.

3. If wandering is attempted in either direction and fails, the forceps must be removed and the entire procedure carefully reassessed. Failure in insertion of the forceps requires consideration of either a trial of vacuum extraction or a resort to cesarean delivery.

Correction of Deflection

1. The fetal head is commonly deflexed in occiput transverse and posterior positions. The obstetric importance of deflection is that the nonflexed fetal head presents a larger diameter to the pelvis than if flexion was present (see Figs. 2.18 and 2.19). Generally deflection is easily corrected as is shown in the following illustration of a fetus in right occiput transverse position (Fig. 3.22).

2. After forceps are applied the fetal head is flexed *between contractions* by a lateral movement of the forceps handle either to the right (as in this example) or to the left as required. The application is then readjusted once the fetal head has reached the correct position, as some slippage often occurs.

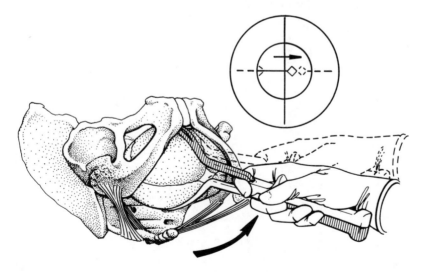

Figure 3.22. ROT position. Correction of cranial deflection. After flexion, the blades are readjusted and rotation is performed, followed by traction.

Correction of Asynclitism

1. In the descent of the fetal head through the midpelvis, arrest disorders are common. In many such instances, the head rotates only partially or not at all from occiput transverse. Depending upon bony pelvic anatomy, tone of pelvic musculature, and the force and consistency of contractions, asynclitism or an oblique presentation of the fetal cranium to the plane of the pelvic curve develops. On palpation the suture line is felt to be curving or bowing either anteriorly (Nägele's obliquity, anterior parietal positions) or posteriorly (Litzmann's obliquity, posterior parietal position), depending upon which parietal bone is presenting (4). Such cranial asymmetry increases the diameter of the fetal cranium and compounds dystocia. Such asynclitism is frequently confusing to the examiner. Particularly with anterior asynclitism, the descent of the fetal head is diagnosed erroneously unless attention is given to the hollow of the sacrum. The posterior pelvis is not filled unless the head is at a low station. Failure of the sacral hollow to be occupied by the fetal head suggests to the surgeon that the true station of the skull is considerably higher than initial palpation of the presenting part suggests. Correction by use of a sliding lock forceps (Barton, or Kielland) is required before progress can continue.

2. With the forceps correctly applied, the operator notes that the handles do not meet correctly due to the cranial malposition (Fig. 3.23). Simultaneously sliding one handle forward and the other backward corrects the presentation and brings the fetal head into the correct orientation to the pelvic outlet (Fig. 3.24).

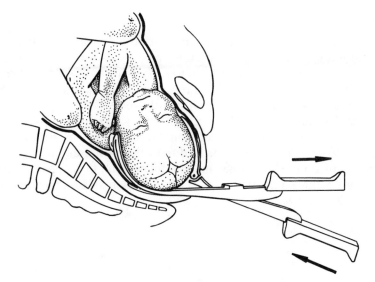

Figure 3.23. LOT position. Anterior asynclitism. Nägele's obliquity, anterior parietal position. Barton forceps applied. Correction indicated.

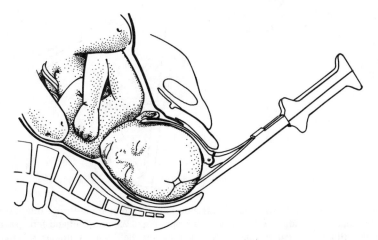

Figure 3.24. LOT position. Correct orientation of fetal head following correction of asynclitism. Barton forceps applied.

Rotation

1. The cardinal principles in rotation are correct application, minimal force, and careful attention to the pelvic curve of the chosen instrument. The greater the pelvic curve, the greater the plane of rotation for the blade handles. The force applied in rotation is closely related to the radius through which handles pass.

2. In the following illustrations, the Kielland, Simpson, and Barton forceps are depicted in rotational operations. The striking difference between the instruments is due to the variations in angle between the plane of the shanks and the blade. Due to its absence of a pelvic curve, the Kielland forceps is often chosen as a midpelvic rotator (Figs. 3.25–3.27).

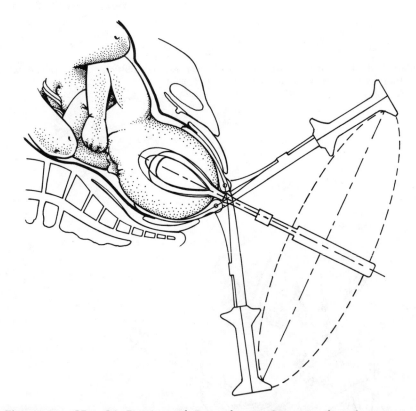

Figure 3.25.   OP to OA. Rotation with Barton forceps. Compare radius of rotation imposed by blade angulation with Simpson forceps (Fig. 3.26) and Kielland forceps (Fig. 3.27). (Modified from Parry-Jones EJ. Barton's forceps. Baltimore: Williams & Wilkins, 1972.)

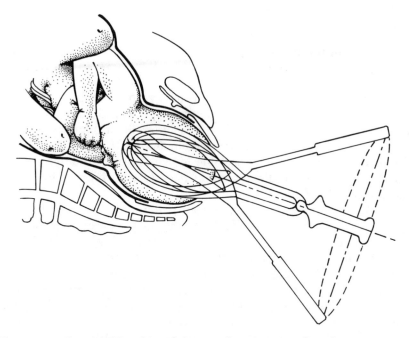

Figure 3.26.   Rotation OP to OA with Simpson forceps. Note radius of rotation imposed by pelvic curve. (Modified from Parry-Jones EJ. Barton's forceps. Baltimore: Williams & Wilkins, 1972.)

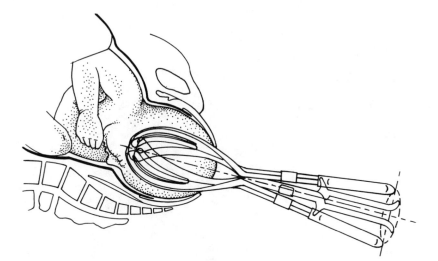

Figure 3.27.   Rotation OP to OA with Kielland forceps. Note radius of rotation. (Modified from Parry-Jones EJ. Barton's forceps. Baltimore: Williams & Wilkins, 1972.)

Application: Special Instruments

Barton Forceps

One of the more unusual forceps in use is the Barton instrument. The blade was initially designed for transverse arrests with the presenting part high in the pelvis. It is particularly useful in the occasional transverse arrest occurring in women with a platypelloid pelvis. But this instrument can be used by an experienced surgeon in any midpelvic transverse arrest. It is much different in application from standard blades and thus harder for the neophyte to learn. Due also to its unusual angulation, it is possible to achieve great rotational force with this instrument and extra care is necessary during rotational maneuvers (see Fig. 3.25).

1. The blades are ghosted against the perineum. The bladder should be emptied by catheterization. The hinged or anterior blade is chosen and held horizontally in the operator's hand with the hollow of the blade directed upward. The blade is inserted posterolaterally in the usual fashion (Fig. 3.28). The blade is then wandered across the fetal face until it reaches its correct position against the anterior fetal parietal bone. As the blade is hinged, an assistant is required to hold the handle in an upward position after it has been applied so the posterior blade can be introduced without obstruction (4, 5, 10, 23).

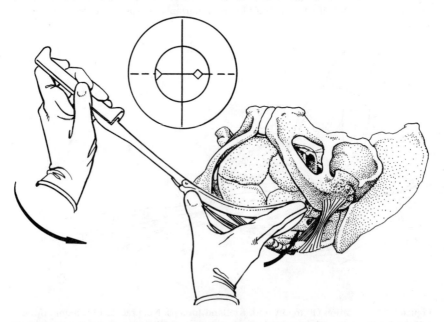

Figure 3.28. ROT. Insertion of the anterior blade of Barton forceps posterolaterally prior to wandering.

2. Uncommonly, if marked anterior asynclitism is present, the anterior blade can be applied directly by simply advancing it progressively from below over the presenting fetal parietal bone. (Note: this application is not illustrated.)

3. The posterior blade is introduced slightly obliquely and to the left of the anterior blade (Fig. 3.29). This application is sometimes moderately difficult. The operator's vaginal hand presses the advancing edge of the blade gently against the fetal head, "rocking" it slowly forward in a technique similar to wandering until it lies fully against the posterior fetal parietal bone.

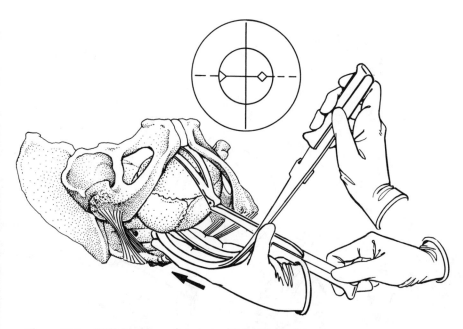

Figure 3.29.   ROT. Insertion of posterior blade, Barton forceps.

4. Once the application is complete, the blades are articulated and cranial asynclitism is corrected as necessary, using the sliding lock (Figs. 3.23 and 3.24). Deflection is also corrected, if present (Fig. 3.22).

5. Traction with Barton forceps is performed either with a special axis traction handle or by a modification of the Saxtorph-Pajot maneuver (Fig. 3.30). Traction is not made in the direction of the handles, as with a more conventional forceps, but in the pelvic axis. If the axis traction handle is not used, the operator's right hand is used simply to stablize and maintain positioning of the two blades of the forceps. The left hand applies the tractive force by grasping the instrument near the lock and pulling in the pelvic curve. With descent of the presenting part, the operator's arms pivot, resulting in the correct vector of force.

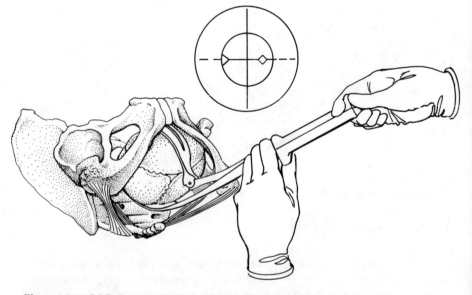

Figure 3.30. ROT. Traction applied to Barton forceps. An axis traction handle or towel-assisted traction can also be used.

6. If an axis traction handle is not available, a towel may be wrapped around the shank of the blade to assist in traction. With either a towel or handle the pull is in the pelvic curve. As the head descends through the birth canal, rotation occurs at the introitus in patients with a platypelloid pelvis and otherwise progressively with traction as the head descends in women with more normal pelvic anatomy (Fig. 3.31). After rotation to OA the Barton forceps may be removed and replaced with a conventional forceps at the operator's discretion. Due to their unusual angulation, the Barton forceps can produce considerable force during rotation and especial care is necessary (see Fig. 3.25).

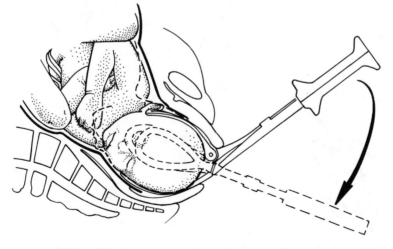

Figure 3.31.   ROT to LOA. Movement of the fetal head and forceps handle with traction, Barton forceps. Final cranial position after rotation is depicted.

Kielland Forceps: Classic Application (Inversion Technique)

1. When Kielland forceps are applied by the classic or inversion technique, the *anterior* blade is inserted first. It is extremely important that the blade be applied *within* the cervix—thus, full dilatation is mandatory. The patient's bladder must be emptied by catheterization to avoid injury.

2. First, the articulated blades are ghosted in front of the perineum, angled to the position they will occupy when correctly applied (Fig. 3.32). Kielland forceps have a button on the finger guard that assists the operator in aligning the anterior blade. The button should always be *toward the occiput* once the blade is applied against the fetal head.

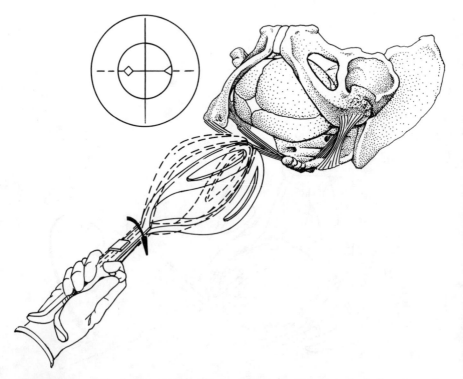

Figure 3.32.   LOT. Ghosting Kielland forceps. The operator orients the buttons toward the occiput.

3. For insertion, the operator's left hand is passed into the vagina palm up with one or more fingers between the cervix and the fetal head. The anterior, right forceps blade is inserted into the vagina with the cephalic curve facing upward. The toe of the blade is passed along the operator's hand to enter the uterus (Fig. 3.33A). *It is particularly important to pass the blade within the cervix and into the uterus.*

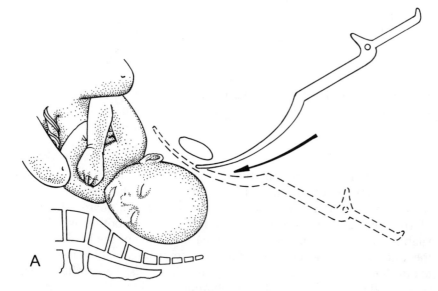

Figure 3.33A.   LOT position. Kielland forceps, inversion technique, initial insertion of anterior (right) blade.

4. The anterior blade is slowly advanced *within the cervix* and under the pubic symphysis until the toe of the blade can be seen to bulge the maternal abdominal wall upward. The blade is advanced with care and must never be forced (4, 5, 7, 20, 22) (Fig. 3.33B).

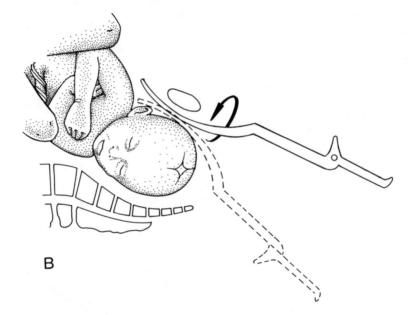

B

Figure 3.33B.   LOT position. Inversion of the anterior blade of Kielland forceps following insertion.

5. Once the anterior blade has reached the correct position with the handle descending below the horizontal, the operator simply rotates the handle of the blade 180° *away from the occiput* between uterine contractions. The forceps should rotate smoothly within the vagina and come to rest with the cephalic hollow of the blade against the anterior fetal parietal bone. Excessive force must not be used. If the blade does not rotate easily, the application must be carefully reassessed. When the blade rotation is completed and the blade is correctly applied, it lies against the fetal parietal bone with the *button toward the occiput*. If the blade is not centered against the parietal bone, it is wandered into the appropriate position.

6. With the anterior blade correctly applied and held by an assistant, the operator then inserts the posterior blade obliquely, taking care to cross the handle of the anterior blade. This ensures easy articulation. The blade is then introduced and wandered into the correct position against the posterior fetal parietal bone (Fig. 3.34). The vaginal hand assists this procedure by "walking" the blade between the vaginal vault and the fetal head.

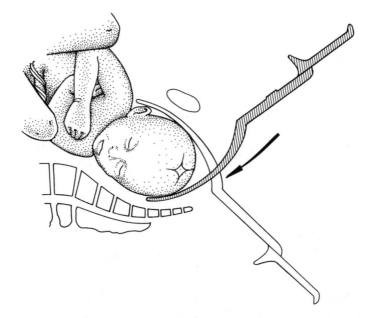

Figure 3.34.   LOT. Kielland forceps, insertion of posterior (left) blade.

7. Kielland forceps can also be applied by the wandering technique. In this procedure, the anterior blade is inserted posterolaterally in the same fashion as previously described for the application of a classic forceps to the OA position (Fig. 3.35).

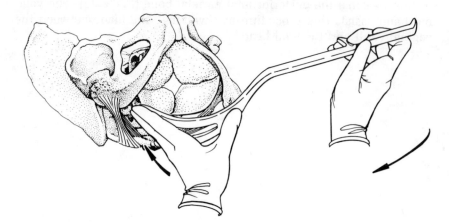

Figure 3.35.   LOT. Kielland forceps. Introduction of (right) anterior blade for wandering application.

8. Once inserted, the blade is then progressively wandered across the fetal face until it reaches its final position against the parietal bone (Fig. 3.36). Insertion of the posterior blade follows. Due to ease

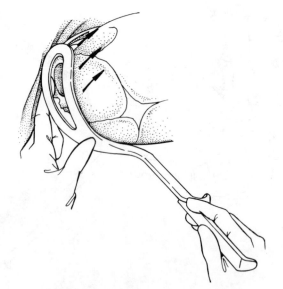

Figure 3.36.   LOT. Kielland forceps. Wandering of (right) anterior blade.

of application, the wandering technique is favored by many clinicians.

9. Some operators, however, prefer *direct application*. In this technique, the toe of the anterior blade is applied against the fetal head with the cephalic curve down. The blade is progressively advanced along the side of the fetal head until it reaches the correct position. To achieve its final position, the blade is "walked" or wandered slowly along the fetal head assisted by the vaginal hand. Generally, this technique only works if marked anterior cranial asynclitism is present. (Note: this application is not illustrated.)

10. When the blades are correctly applied, the attitude of the fetal head is corrected for deflection and asynclitism (Fig. 3.37). Refer also to Figs. 3.22–3.24.

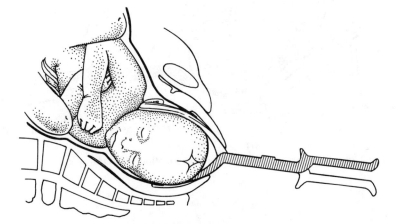

Figure 3.37.   LOT. Kielland forceps. Cranial deflection and asynclitism are corrected prior to rotation. The buttons are toward the occiput.

11. Midpelvic rotation is then performed (Fig. 3.38). Rotation should be easy and is generally performed with one hand, using gentle pressure. Frequently, the fetal head may need to be displaced to a slightly higher station in order to permit rotation. Note the narrow radius of rotation imposed by the absent pelvic curve (see Fig. 3.27).

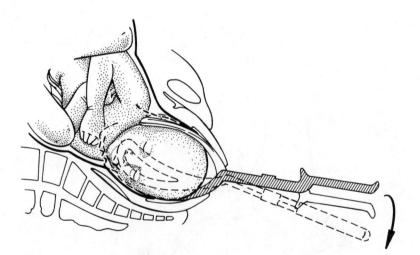

Figure 3.38. LOT position. Kielland forceps. Rotation LOT-OA.

12. Traction by the Saxtorph-Pajot maneuver is applied once rotation is complete (Fig. 3.39). As Kielland forceps have no pelvic curve, the plane of shank of the articulated blades must *never* be raised above the plane of the midpelvis, or else the toe of the blade will impinge upon the posterior vaginal tissues, resulting in serious maternal lacerations (4, 35). Some operators prefer to replace the Kielland forceps by a classic blade for traction/delivery.

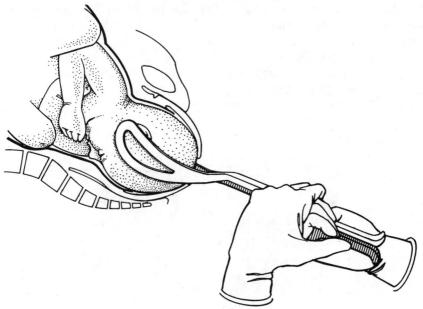

Figure 3.39.   Traction, Kielland forceps.

Special Applications

Aftercoming Head (Breech Presentation): Piper Forceps

The most important special application is the application of forceps to the head of the aftercoming breech. While a number of forceps have been described for use in this position, the most popular has been the instrument originally described by Piper. The Piper forceps is a long, flexible instrument that is used to maintain the position of the fetal head and attempt to avoid complications of fetal intracranial injury during breech delivery (36).

This application is the only *pelvic* as opposed to *cephalic* forceps operation. The blades of the Piper forceps are introduced in the same fashion for all deliveries.

1. The operator delivers the child to the umbilicus. An assistant supports the infant's body with either a hand or towel (Fig. 3.40). The baby is moved laterally toward the mother's right to ease the blade insertion. The operator inserts the blades from below. Crouching or kneeling to achieve the correct angle for insertion, the left blade is always inserted first. The accoucheur applies the *left* blade of the forceps alongside the *right* parietal bone of the fetal head. During the insertion, the handle of the blade is swept upward and toward the operator's right. The surgeon's right hand enters the vagina to assist this insertion, guiding the blade's advance along the left side of the vaginal canal with gentle but firm digital pressure.

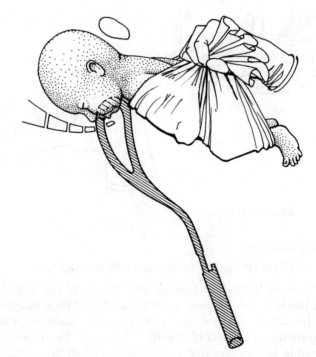

Figure 3.40.   Breech presentation. Insertion of *left* blade. Piper forceps.

2. With the left blade introduced, the infant's body is moved toward the mother's left to assist in the application of the right blade. The second or *right* blade is then introduced with care to overlap the left blade, facilitating articulation when the insertion is complete (4, 5, 36, 37) (Fig. 3.41).

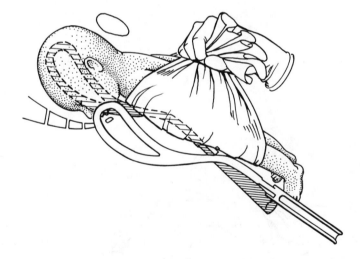

Figure 3.41.   Breech presentation. Insertion of *right* blade. Piper forceps.

3. When the application is complete, the blades are articulated. The operator's *right* hand controls the forceps, grasping the finger hold and maintaining opposition of the flexible blades. Usually it is convenient to grasp one or both of the infant's legs to better stabilize the body. The surgeon's *left* hand lies along the fetal back and alongside the fetal neck at the occiput for support. Traction is then applied in the pelvic curve with careful attention not to raise the plane of the forceps above the horizontal until the head is passing through the introitus. Especially with smaller infants care is taken to be certain that the baby's head does not fall from between the flexible blades of the forceps after extraction (Fig. 3.42).

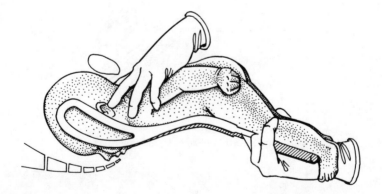

Figure 3.42.   Breech presentation. Traction. Piper forceps.

Occiput Posterior (OP) or Oblique Positions

The application of forceps or the vacuum extractor to the occiput posterior position is controversial. Historically, opinions have varied from a position of favoring prompt operative intervention (37) to a *laissez faire* attitude of watchful expectancy (38). There is genuine concern over posterior positions, due to their strong association with dystocia and fetal heart rate abnormalities. Careful analysis of data on the progress of labor in patients with posterior presentations indicates an increased frequency of uterine tachysystole, hypertonia, and tetanic contraction (39). Further, electronic fetal heart rate tracings are more likely to be abnormal in these patients than in similar women with anterior presentations (40). Variable-type decelerations are particularly common. It is speculated that the increased frequency of variable fetal heart rate decelerations is secondary to increased fetal cranial or intratracheal compression/pressure, with a corresponding increase in vagal tone (40).

In the past it was held that posterior presentations were pathologic and rotation to an anterior presentation was indicated. Today, feelings about occiput posterior presentations are mixed (19, 34). Some clinicians will deliver a posterior presentation directly, face to pubis by forceps without an attempt at rotation. Vacuum extraction is also possible and is discussed in Chapter 4 (24). Principal forceps rotational operations from the direct OP or oblique posterior positions are by (a) the modified Scanzoni maneuver; (b) the reverse Scanzoni maneuver, using a classic forceps; or (c) direct application of Kielland forceps.

The incidence of occiput posterior positioning in early labor is estimated at approximately 20% (Table 3.5) with a range from 13 to 30%, depending upon the series. Spontaneous rotation during the

Table 3.5. Incidence of Occipitoposterior (OP) Position, Selected Series

Author	Total N	Percent overall Incidence OP	Percent Persistent OP[a]
Dodek (41)	1,785	29.9% (514)	
Danforth (42)	1,137	25.1% (285)	
Lull (43)	927	22.1% (204)	
Scott (44)	1,000	14.4% (144)	
Reddoch (45)	948	19.5% (185)	
Kutchipal (46)	5,396		9.3% (498)
Cannell (15)	1,817	13.4% (244)	5.9% (107)
Phillips & Freedman (47)	8,120		6.8% (552)
Sokol et al. (39)	380	13.7% (52)	
Ingemarsson et al. (40)	3,098		4.5% (138)
Total	24,608	20.4% (1628/7994)	7.1% (1,295/18,431)

[a]Failure to spontaneously rotate to a transverse or anterior position during labor.

progress of labor reduces the incidence to 7.1% at the time of actual delivery. Occiput posterior positions are more uncomfortable for both physician and patient, and numerous schemes of management have been suggested (Table 3.6).

Table 3.6. Management Options for Occiput Posterior/Oblique Positions

Nonoperative
  Watchful expectancy (38)
  Maternal repositioning (Puddicombe's maneuver) (48)
Operative
  Manual rotation (33)
    Simple rotation (15)
    Holland maneuver (16)
    Pomeroy-Lackie maneuver (17–19)
  Delivery OP
    Forceps (34)
    Vacuum (24)
  Barton forceps rotation (33)
  Kielland rotation (20, 21, 49)
  Modified Scanzoni rotation (37, 45, 50, 51)
  Reverse Scanzoni (single application) (19, 52, 53)
  Haas maneuver (Scanzoni without blade reversal) (46)
  Key-in-lock maneuver (54)
  Modified manual-Laufe rotation (55)
  Single blade (manual-vectis) rotation, Merchan's maneuver (56)
  Single blade (vectis rotation), Maughan's maneuver (57)

The majority of posterior positions occur in women with gynecoid-type pelves. However, certain variations in pelvic architecture predispose to this presentation (Table 3.7). A shortened transverse diameter (anthropoid/android tendency), narrow forepelvis, prominent ischial spines, straight sacrum, or convergent side walls increase the likelihood that the occiput will enter the hind pelvis preferentially. There is some unique constellation of factors involving mild abnormalities of pelvic structure combined with features of the maternal

Table 3.7. Predisposing Factors for Occiput Posterior (OP) Positioning[a]

Maternal
  Multiparity/laxity of abdominal wall and uterus
  Pelvic abnormality
    Narrow forepelvis
    Prominent ischial spine
    Convergent side walls
    Shortened transverse diameter
  Prior OP delivery
  (?) Conduction anesthesia
Fetal
  Deflection of fetal head
  Brachycephaly

[a]See Refs. 33, 45, and 46.

abdominal wall or uterine tone that results in a 40% recurrence risk for posterior positioning in women who experience subsequent pregnancies (46). Regional anesthesia is also implicated in persistent posterior positions. Presumably, relaxation of pelvic musculature interferes with spontaneous cranial rotation. However, it is unclear whether cranial deflection and poor uterine contractions are the cause or the result of posterior positioning (33, 38, 39). In any event, 70–75% of initially posterior presentations will spontaneously rotate to the anterior. Thus, poor uterine contractions are not a factor in most instances. Interestingly, the incidence of right occiput posterior (ROP) is 3–5-fold greater than the corresponding left occiput posterior (LOP) position (42). Presumably dextrorotation of the uterus and the presence of the rectosigmoid colon in the left lower quadrant deny the left posterior position to the fetus (33).

Normally, anterior rotation of the occiput does not occur until after complete cervical dilatation. Thus, expectancy is the rule in early labor (37). When to consider intervention is controversial at best. The rule for occiput posterior presentations should be the same as with anterior presentations. No intervention is indicated in the face of a normal mother and fetus until progress ceases. If progress is arrested, the attendant may attempt Puddicombe's maneuver, placing the woman in knee-chest position to hasten rotation (48). The effectiveness of such postural management is difficult to evaluate, as 75% of posterior presentations will rotate to the anterior without any special maneuvers (33). However, nothing is lost and perhaps there can be some gain by placing the mother in either the knee-chest or modified Sim's position to assist spontaneous rotation. Theoretically, repositioning assists the forces of gravity in promoting rotation. Alternatively, repositioning can displace the fetal body away from the maternal spine, changing the orientation of the fetal mass in the maternal abdomen, altering body or head position. If positioning proves impossible or unavailing, then manual rotation or instrumental assistance is attempted.

The infant may be delivered simply as an OP (face to pubis) although the pull can be difficult (34, 35). In delivery face to pubis, the forceps are applied as to the corresponding anterior presentation and thus are "upside down" on the fetal head (Fig. 3.43). Thus, in a reversal of the usual application, the *left* forceps blade lies along the *right* side of the fetal head, the *right* blade along the *left*. As deflection is common, the head is flexed *anteriorly* before traction is attempted. When correctly applied, the forceps will be oriented in the midline one finger breadth *above* the posterior fontanelle. Traction is made posteriorly until the fetal forehead passes beneath the pubic symphysis. The head is then slowly extracted by flexion. Since flexion is limited and the greatest bulk of the fetal head is posterior, an episiotomy is necessary and extensions are common.

Manual rotation may be tried but is not commonly successful. However, finger splinted or spontaneous rotation accompanying vacuum extraction may work (24, 25). Two variants of manual rotation involving forceps deserve comment: the modified *manual-Laufe rotation of Goodlin* (55) and the single blade or *vectis rotation of Merchan* (56). In both, a forceps blade (or blades) assists manual rotation of the fetal head. The aim is to avoid fetal/maternal injuries due to blade manipulation.

The *vectis rotation of Maughan* (57) is similar except that a simple forceps blade is introduced upside down to the opposite side of the maternal pelvis then swept across the fetal occiput, catching the anterior fetal ear and rotating it to transverse or beyond (34).

If delivery as an occiput posterior proves unacceptably difficult, or manual or modified manual rotations fail, then anterior forceps rotation is attempted. The best known technique for delivery of posterior positions is the Scanzoni rotation or its modifications (Table 3.6). These procedures are not for the inexperienced. Approximately·25% of neonates subjected to major rotations exhibit discrete, transient neurological signs. Fortunately these resolve spontaneously within a week generally without any sequelae (58). In frank fetal distress or if any difficulty develops during the forceps operation, cesarean section is often the best management.

The *Scanzoni maneuver*, as generally described, is that modified by Bill (37) and Seides (59) from the original description of Scanzoni/Smellie (5). In brief, a forceps—usually a Tucker-McLane, but any outlet-type blade is acceptable—is applied *upside down* as if to the corresponding anterior position (Figs. 3.44 and 3.45). That is, an OP is considered as a OA, a LOP as a ROP, etc. Once the application is completed and cranial deflection corrected, the fetal head is rotated to OA, *without traction* (Fig. 3.46, A and B).

The posterior forceps blade is left *in situ* and the anterior blade removed. A second forceps blade is then reintroduced alongside the splinting blade with the convex portion of the blade correctly oriented toward the fetal occiput (Figs. 3.47–3.49). That is, the second blade is applied "right side up." The splinting blade is then removed and the remaining blade of the second forceps introduced. Following rechecking of the application and corrections of deflection, traction is made and delivery accomplished (35, 34, 37).

A number of variations of this technique exist. As removal and reinsertion of the blades risk fetal/maternal injury and/or loss of station, several maneuvers are described to achieve delivery using the *initally* inserted blade for delivery. In this, the so-called *reverse Scanzoni maneuver*, the blades are initially inserted *correctly oriented for the posterior occiput* (Fig. 3.51). In this procedure, the handle position of the forceps is the *reverse* of the usual orientation as the shanks will point *downward*. Thus, particular care is necessary during flexion and rotation. The rotation is made to OA or slightly oblique, the application rechecked, and traction for delivery made without replacing or reversing the blades (19, 52, 53). In the *Haas maneuver*, the blades are initially applied as for a regular Scanzoni but after rotation are *not removed*. The fetal head is simply delivered using the upside down forceps (46). *The DeLee lock-in-key procedure* with its multiple forceps reapplications is of historic interest only (4, 54).

In the *Kielland rotation*, the blades are ghosted as for the corresponding *anterior* application (Fig. 3.52). That is, an ROP is initially considered as an LOA, an OP as an OA, etc. The blades are then rotated 180° and thus appear upside down to the operator but are correctly aligned with the fetal occiput. Direct application *from below* follows. With the blades correctly introduced, the fetal head is flexed and rotated anteriorly. After rotation, the forceps alignment is then rechecked prior to traction/delivery. As the Kielland is an indifferent traction forceps, some operators replace it with a classic outlet-type blade for delivery.

Instrumental rotation from occiput posterior to anterior is easiest performed using Kielland forceps. Experienced operators may try the Scanzoni rotation, as modified by Bill; however, *Bill's procedure is not recommended for the neophyte without close and expert instruction.* Posterior to anterior rotations can generate remarkable vaginal lacerations in unskilled hands.

Occiput Posterior (OP) Position: Delivery as an OP, Face to Pubis

1. The blades are ghosted and applied as for the corresponding *anterior* presentation (Fig. 3.43). Thus, a direct OP is handled as an OA, the ROP as an LOA, etc. Once applied, the pull is longer and usually more difficult than the corresponding OA position and rectal extensions are common. As the posterior head cannot deliver by extension, the posterior force on the perineum is substantial. The operator must pull posteriorly until the forehead, orbits, and then cheeks of the infant appear before he/she can take advantage of the slight degree of cranial flexion possible on the perineum. The fetal head is commonly *deflexed* in posterior presentations. Flexion by anterior manipulation of the blades is appropriate to present the birth canal with the smallest possible cranial diameter (34).

2. An axis traction handle may assist this operation.

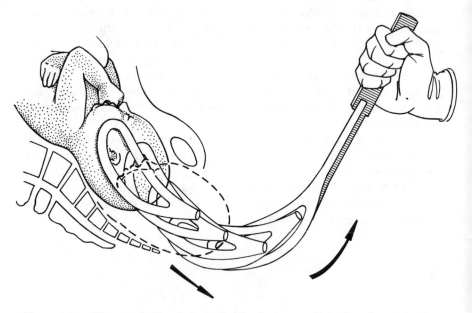

Figure 3.43. OP presentation. Delivery by classic forceps. Note direction of traction with delivery of the head by flexion (34).

Occiput Posterior or Oblique Position: Modified Scanzoni Rotation

1. Bill's modification of the Scanzoni maneuver requires either two pairs of forceps or a reintroduction of the blades of the initial set. Forceps are ghosted and applied to the posterior position as if it were the corresponding anterior presentation (Figs. 3.44 and 3.45). Thus, once applied, the forceps are upside down for the fetal occiput (4, 5, 15, 17, 37, 45, 50, 51, 59).

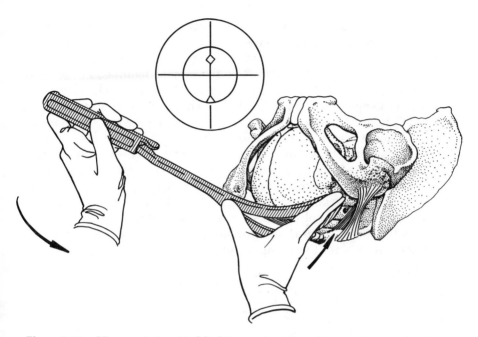

Figure 3.44.   OP presentation. Modified Scanzoni rotation. Simpson forceps. Application of left forceps blade.

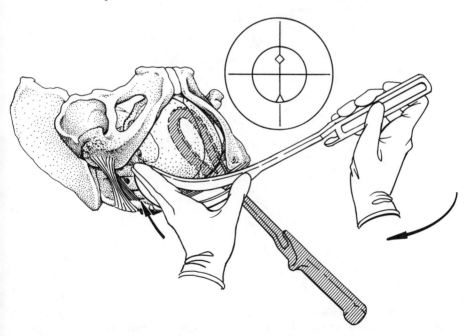

Figure 3.45.   OP presentation. Modified Scanzoni rotation. Simpson forceps. Application of right forceps blade.

2. The blades are articulated. Rotation to the anterior position, usually with some overcorrection, follows (Fig. 3.46, A and B). Rotation must be performed with great care if a classic forceps is used. A wide arc is necessarily inscribed by the forceps handles, imposed by the pelvic curve. When such a blade has been applied, during the rotation the operator should "push the handles to the thighs" (see Fig. 3.26). Care must be taken to maintain the angle between the plane of the perineum and that of the shanks of the blades constant, or else serious maternal laceration may occur. When rotation is completed, one forceps blade is then removed, with the *posterior* blade left to splint the fetal head, preventing rerotation to the original position. The forceps are then reapplied "correctly," the adjustments checked, and tractions to achieve delivery performed. Note that at the completion of the rotation the occiput is *anterior* but the blades appear upside down to the operator with the shanks now pointing toward the floor.

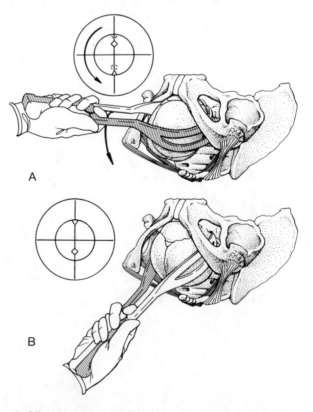

A

B

Figure 3.46. *A*, OP presentation. Modified Scanzoni rotation. Simpson forceps. Rotation OP to OA. Note at completion of the rotation the forceps shanks point *down. B*, OP presentation. Modified Scanzoni rotation. Forceps orientation at completion of posterior to anterior rotation.

3. One forceps blade is then removed, with the *posterior* blade left to splint the fetal head, preventing rerotation to the original position (Fig. 3.47). The forceps are then reapplied correctly. Either the original forceps may be used or, as is shown here, a second pair may be inserted. Due to the position of the blades and the pelvic curve, the forceps are removed from below, in a sweeping motion following the cephalic curve of the blade.

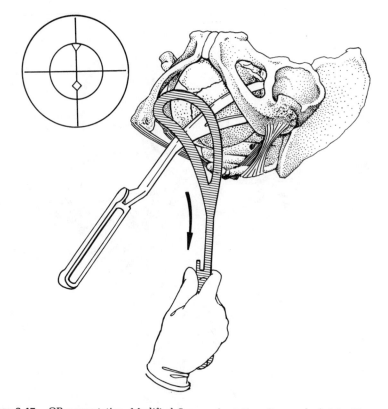

Figure 3.47. OP presentation. Modified Scanzoni rotation. Removal of right Simpson forceps blade. Left blade splints the fetal head.

4. A second forceps application is now made (Figs. 3.48 and 3.49). The second application is simply the classic OA application with the left blade inserted to the left side of the fetal head in the OA or LOA position. As is depicted here the new blade can be inserted inside the splinting blade. Alternatively the companion blade—here the right blade—can be inserted on the opposite side of the fetal head to avoid any difficulties with blade interaction. Once the new blade is inserted, the splinting blade is removed from below.

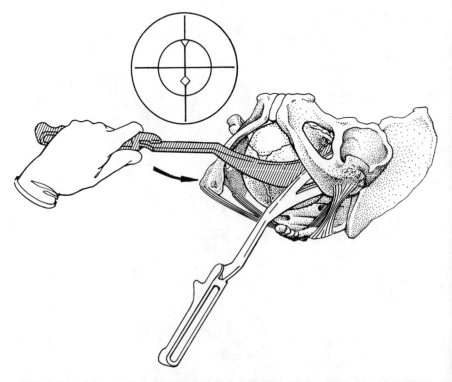

Figure 3.48. OP presentation. Modified Scanzoni rotation. Insertion left blade Tucker-McLane forceps.

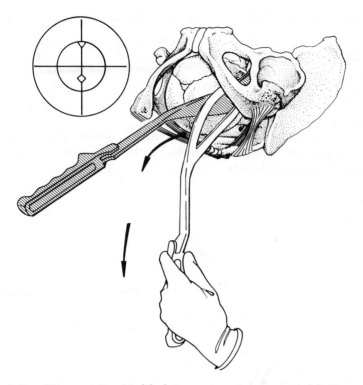

Figure 3.49. OP presentation. Modified Scanzoni rotation. Removal right Simpson forceps blade.

5. The newly inserted blades are articulated, the application checked, and any adjustments are made (Fig. 3.50). Traction for delivery follows.

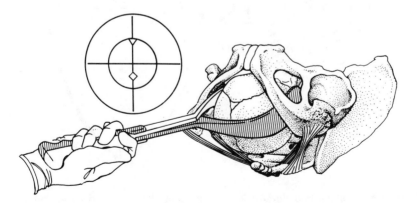

Figure 3.50. OP presentation. Modified Scanzoni rotation. Tucker-McLane forceps applied to OA head after rotation and reinsertion.

Occiput Posterior or Oblique Position: Reverse Scanzoni Rotation

1. In this procedure the forceps are correctly applied to the fetal head in posterior position (Fig. 3.51). *They thus appear upside down to the operator as the handles point toward the floor.*

2. The angulation of the blades requires that they be introduced from *below* the horizontal plane, in a mirror image of a standard OA application.

3. The head is flexed by *downward* motion. Rotation to OA follows. Great care must be taken due to the unfamiliar angulation of the forceps during this maneuver (see Fig. 3.26) (19).

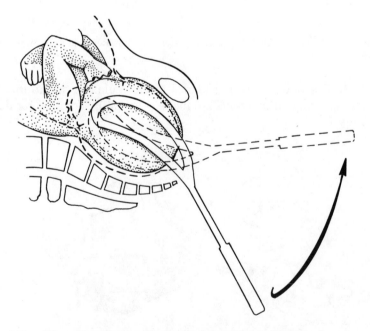

Figure 3.51.   OP position. Reverse Scanzoni rotation OP-OA. (Redrawn from Savage JE. Forceps delivery. Clin Obstet Gynecol 1958;4:917–939).

Occiput Posterior or Oblique Position: Kielland Forceps

1. The blades are first ghosted for their application (Fig. 3.52). The blades are initially oriented as for an OA position then *reversed 180° with the buttons toward the occiput.*

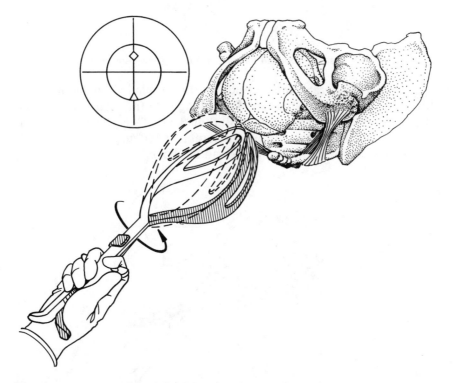

Figure 3.52.   OP position. Kielland forceps. Ghosting of forceps.

2. The blades are inserted from below, with the angle of insertion governed by the slight pelvic curve of the instrument (Fig. 3.53). In the direct OP either blade can be inserted first; however, it is most convenient to insert the right blade first to facilitate locking. In posterior oblique positions (ROP, LOP) the posterior or right blade is applied first, followed by the left or anterior blade. The anterior blade can be directly applied as shown. Alternatively, the anterior blade is inserted posterolaterally in the usual manner and wandered into the correct position (4).

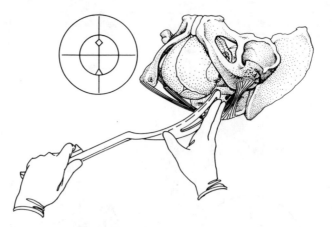

Figure 3.53. OP position. Kielland forceps, insertion of posterior or right branch.

3. The operator then introduces the left blade from below using his/her left hand to swing the blade along side the fetal head against the right maternal vaginal side wall (Fig. 3.54). This procedure is simply the application to an OA position, rotated 180° and performed with the blades coming from *below* instead of above.

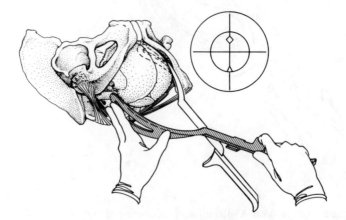

Figure 3.54. ROP position. Kielland forceps, insertion of anterior or left branch.

4. The application is now checked and the head flexed if necessary. As always, the buttons are *toward the occiput*. With the application correct, the handle of the blades is swept 180° to rotate the fetal head to OA (Fig. 3.55). Care must be taken to maintain the angle between the plane of the perineum and that of the shanks of the blades constant, or else serious maternal lacerations may occur.

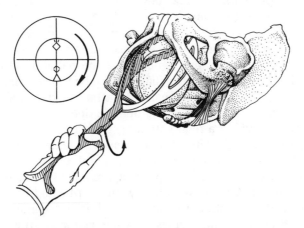

Figure 3.55.   OP posterior. Kielland forceps. Rotation OP to OA.

5. With the head at OA position, the application is rechecked and, if necessary, readjusted (Fig. 3.56). Once rotation is complete some operators will remove the Kielland forceps and apply a classic outlet blade. However, the Kielland forceps may be used as long as care is taken with traction to avoid elevation of the shanks above the horizontal.

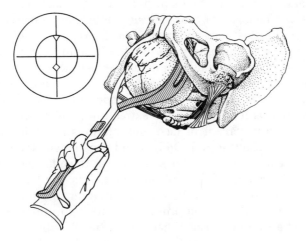

Figure 3.56.   OP posterior. Kielland forceps. Rotation OP to OA complete.

Brow and Face Presentations

Extreme cranial deflection results in either brow or face presentation. Such abnormalities in presentation are uncommon, occurring at a rate of approximately 2.2/1000 deliveries and provide unique challenges for the obstetrician.

Face presentation is more common in multiparas than in nulliparas. Most face presentations are a secondary extension taking place during the process of labor, generally at the pelvic inlet (34).

Brow presentation is usually felt to be transitional between full flexion to vertex or full extension to a face. Extension attitudes are commonly associated with cephalopelvic disproportion. Thus, a relatively small pelvis or a relatively large head must be carefully considered in the etiology. Uncommon causes of extension include fetal anencephaly, cystic hygroma, thyroid neoplasia, or multiple coils of cord around the neck which prevent flexion (34, 60, 61). However, many instances occur in apparently uncomplicated cases (62). Other possible etiologic factors, including low lying placenta, tumors of the pelvis, hydramnios, and increased extensive tone of the fetal back and neck muscles, have also been supported or suggested in various reviews. Brow presentations are usually transitional and may convert spontaneously to a face or occiput posterior. However, the likelihood of spontaneous delivery of a brow is low, only about 10% (63). If a brow is present and any suggestion of disproportion exists, cesarean section should be performed. The uncommon brow that will deliver vaginally presents as a mentum anterior with the occiput in the hollow of the sacrum. Use of the forceps in brow presentation is uncommonly indicated. The instrument of choice is Kielland forceps with the directional markers oriented to the posterior fontanelle. Once the blades are applied, the majority of brow presentations can be converted by flexion to occiput posterior and rotated or delivered as a direct posterior. When applied to the anterior brow, the Kielland forceps are inverted with the anterior fontanelle lying just beneath the plane of the shanks with the directional markers oriented toward the posterior fontanelle. Once applied, an attempt should be made to flex the head to an occiput posterior as it will make the extraction much easier.

Seventy percent of face presentations are anterior transverse and 30% are posterior (64). On Leopold's maneuver a marked cephalic prominence is palpated on the same side as the fetal back and, depending upon the extent of descent into the pelvis, the mass palpated can be substantial in size. On pelvic examination, the presenting part is soft and irregular and often initially confusing to the clinician due to edema. The mouth can at times be confused with the anus but the characteristic feel of the maxillar and mandibular ridges and palpation of the orbits should clinch the diagnosis. Occasionally the fetus may suck the operator's examining finger (65). In certain cases, real time ultrasound can exclude breech and may directly confirm the diagnosis.

The mechanism of face delivery requires the mentum to be anterior. The fetal head is delivered in extension until the chin passes beneath the pubic symphysis. Thereafter, the remainder of the head is then delivered by flexion. Labor characteristically is longer in face presentation. With the process of labor and with maternal pushing the fetal face frequently becomes markedly edematous. Rarely, edema of the larynx may result from prolonged pressure of the hyoid region against the pubic bone and result in neonatal respiratory problems.

The best management for face presentation is watchful expectancy (60). Manual attempts at rotation are usually unavailing. As long as progress is being made and the fetal heart tracing is acceptable, no intervention is indicated. The majority of face presentations will rotate to anterior and deliver spontaneously (66). If the mentum remains a transverse or posterior, cesarean section is best. Uncommonly, in mentum anterior positions forceps may be used. Kielland forceps are recommended for this application but classic forceps may also be used. Because the presentation is unusual the orientation of the blades to the fetal head is different. If classic forceps were used, the mentum replaces the occiput for orientation. If Kielland forceps are applied, the directional indicators are inserted so that they point toward the chin. The blades, when correctly inserted, are level with the supraorbital ridges and the fetal mouth and nose are at the level of the shanks. Once the blades are correctly inserted, the handles are depressed toward the floor to deflex the head completely. Traction is made in a horizontal and slightly posterior direction until the chin appears under the pubic symphysis. As the face and forehead appear, the direction of traction is changed to outward and anterior and both descent and flexion occur. As the largest delivery diameter is posterior, episiotomy extensions and vaginal lacerations are common. Care must be taken with the Kielland forceps not to raise the plane of the forceps above that of the horizontal, or else the heel of the blades will impinge on the posterior vaginal wall, producing remarkable lacerations. In the application of blades, the left forceps blade is applied to the right fetal ear. The left held in the left hand is inserted in the left side of the vagina over the child's right ear. The right blade held in the right hand is inserted over the right side of the vagina over the child's left ear. The application is then checked, using the mouth as a landmark, and replaced with the posterior fontanelle. It is important that complete extension of the head be maintained until the chin is born under the pubic symphysis. The same contraindications for Kielland forceps in occiput presentations apply for the face in either a flat pelvis or flat sacrum shortening of the anterior/posterior diameter of the pelvis, and Kielland forceps should not be used due to the risk of posterior impingement and lacerations (4, 5).

Face Presentation Mentum Anterior: Kielland Forceps

1. Note the special orientation for face presentation (Fig. 3.57). The indicator buttons are *toward* the chin. The fetal mouth and nose lie in the plane of the shanks when the blades are correctly applied. Prior to traction the fetal head must be fully *extended* to present the smallest possible diameter to the pelvis.

2. Traction is made in a slightly posterior direction to maintain cranial extension. The handles of Kielland forceps must never rise above the horizontal. As the head is extracted, delivery is by slow extension until the chin passes beneath the pubic symphysis.

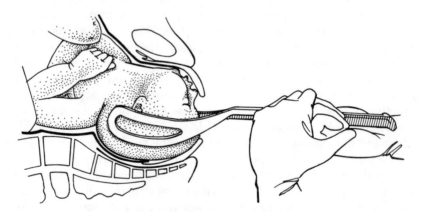

Figure 3.57.   Face presentation. Kielland forceps. Traction to the mentum anterior.

REFERENCES

1. Smellie W. A collection of cases and observations in midwifery. 6th ed. London: 1774.
2. Pajot CP. Travaux d'obstetrique et de gynécologie précédés d'élements de practique obstétricale. Paris: H Lauwereynes, 1882.
3. Mines JL. Application of the obstetric forceps. Obstet Gynecol 1970; 36:680–685.
4. Dennon EH. Forceps deliveries. 2nd ed. Philadelphia: FA Davis, 1964.
5. Laufe LE. Obstetric forceps. New York: Harper & Row, 1968.
6. Pritchard JA, MacDonald PC, Gant NF. Williams obstetrics, 17th ed. Norwalk, Appleton-Century-Crofts, 1985.
7. Martius G. Operative obstetrics, 17th ed. New York: Thieme-Stratton, 1980.
8. Dill LV. The obstetrical forceps. Springfield, Illinois: Charles C Thomas, 1953.

9. Bowes WA, Bowes, C. Current role of the midforceps operation. Clin Obstet Gynecol 1980; 23:549–557.
10. Ahnquist, G. Delivery of the persistent transverse vertex utilizing Barton forceps. W J Surg Obstet Gynecol 1952; 60:406–424.
11. Healy DL, Quinn MA, Pepperell RJ. Rotational delivery of the fetus: Kielland's forceps and two other methods compared. Br J Obstet Gynaecol 1982; 89:501–509.
12. Chiswick ML, James DK. Kielland's forceps: association with neonatal morbidity and mortality. Br Med J 1979; 1:7–9.
13. O'Driscoll K, Foley M, MacDonald D. Active management of labor as an alternative to cesarean section for dystocia. Obstet Gynecol 1984; 63:485–490.
14. Danforth. Transverse arrest. Clin Obstet Gynecol 1965; 8:854–867.
15. Cannell DE. The management of the occiput posterior: use of the Bill-Scanzoni maneuver. Am J Obstet Gynecol 1950; 60:496–504.
16. Holland E, Bourne A. British obstetric and gynaecological practice. Philadelphia: FA Davis, 1955.
17. Willson JR. Atlas of obstetric technique, 2nd ed. St Louis, CV Mosby, 1969.
18. Cochran GC. The Pomeroy maneuver (rotary version). Brooklyn Hosp J 1939–1940; 1–2:155–168.
19. Savage JE. Forceps delivery. Clin Obstet Gynecol 1958; 4:917–939.
20. Jarcho J. The Kielland obstetrical forceps and its application. Am J Obstet Gynecol 1925; 10:35–49.
21. Greenhill JP. The Kielland forceps. Am J Obstet Gynecol 1924; 7:349–464.
22. Kielland C. Uber die anlegung der zange am nicht rotierten kopf mit beschreibung eines neuen zangenmodelles und einer neuen anlegungsmethode. Monatssch Geburtsh Gynakol 1916; 43:48–78.
23. Parry-Jones EJ. Barton's forceps. Baltimore: Williams & Wilkins, 1972.
24. Chalmers JA. The ventouse: the obstetric vacuum extractor. Chicago: Year Book, 1971.
25. Broekuizen FF, Washington JM, Johnson F, Hamilton PR. Vacuum extraction versus forceps delivery: indication and complications, 1979 to 1984. Obstet Gynecol 1987; 69:338–342.
26. Parry-Jones EJ. Barton's forceps its use in transverse position of the fetal head. J Obstet Gynaecol Br Commonw 1968; 75:892–902.
27. Marin RD. A review of the use of Barton's forceps for the rotation of the fetal head from the transverse position. Aust NZ J Obstet Gynaecol 1978; 18:234–237.
28. O'Driscoll K, Meagher D, MacDonald D, Geoghegan F. Traumatic intracranial haemorrhage in first born infants and delivery with obstetric forceps. Br J Obstet Gynaecol 1981; 88:577–581.
29. Traub AI, Morrow RJ, Ritche JWK, Dornan KJ. A continuing use for Kielland's forceps? Br J Obstet Gynaecol 1984; 91:894–898.
30. Drife JO. Kielland or cesarean? Br Med J 1983; 287:309–310.
31. Cardozo LD, Gibb DMF, Studd JWW, Cooper DJ. Should we abandon Kielland forceps? Br Med J 1983; 287:315–317.
32. Nielsen TF, Hokegard FH. Cesarean section and intraoperative surgical complications. Acta Obstet Gynecol Scand 1984; 63:103–108.
33. Anderson DG. Arrested occiput posterior positions. Clin Obstet Gynecol 1965; 8:867–881.
34. Oxorn H. Human labor and birth. 4th ed. New York: Appleton-Century-Crofts, 1980.
35. Russell KP, Frankel IV. Forceps in common use. Clin Obstet Gynecol 1965; 8:822–833.
36. Piper EB, Bachman C. The prevention of fetal injuries in breech delivery. JAMA 1929; 92:217–221.
37. Bill AH. The treatment of the vertex occipito-posterior position. Am J Obstet Gynecol 1931; 22:615–625.
38. Calkins LA. Occiput posterior presentation. Obstet Gynecol 1953; 1:466–471.
39. Sokol RJ, Roux JF, McCarthy S. Computer diagnosis of labor progression: VI. Fetal stress and labor in the occipitoposterior position. Am J Obstet Gynecol 1975; 122:253–260.
40. Ingemarsson E, Ingemarsson I, Solum T, Westgren M. Influence of occiput posterior position on the fetal heart

rate pattern. Obstet Gynecol 1980; 55:301–304.
41. Dodek SM. The vertex posterior position. JAMA 1931; 96:1660–1664.
42. Danforth WC. Treatment of occipitoposterior with especial reference to manual rotation. Am J Obstet Gynecol 1932; 23:360–366.
43. Lull CB. An analysis of 1,000 obstetric case histories. Am J Obstet Gynecol 1933; 24:75–86.
44. Scott RA. Posterior occiput presentations: analytical review of posterior occiput presentation in 1,000 consecutive deliveries at Evanston Hospital. Am J Obstet Gynecol 1932; 23:400–403.
45. Reddoch JW. The management of occipitoposterior positions with special reference to the Scanzoni maneuver. S Med J 1934; 27:615–623.
46. Kutchipal RA. The persistent occiput posterior position: a review of 498 cases. Obstet Gynecol 1959; 14:296–304.
47. Phillips RD, Freedman M. The management of the persistent occiput posterior position: a review of 552 consecutive cases. Obstet Gynecol 1974; 43:171–177.
48. Puddicombe JF. Maternal posture for correction of posterior fetal position. J Int Col Surg 1955; 23:73–77.
49. Cosgrove SA. Occipitoposterior positions. Am J Obstet Gynecol 1936; 31:402–408.
50. Bill AH. Forceps delivery. Am J Obstet Gynecol 1954; 68:245–249.
51. Pieri RJ. The occipitoposterior position and the modified Scanzoni maneuver. NY State J Med 1940; 40:1773–1778.
52. Smith JT. Single application of forceps to correct occipitoposterior position. Am J Obstet Gynecol 1957; 73:947–953.
53. Williamson HC. Clinic of Dr. Hervey

Clock Williamson: the use and abuse of forceps. Surg Clin North Am 1935; 15:513–525.
54. DeLee JB. Treatment of occiput posterior position after engagement of the head. Surg Gynecol Obstet 1928; 46:696–700.
55. Goodlin RC. Modified manual rotation in pelvic delivery. Obstet Gynecol 1986; 67:128–130.
56. Merchan RR. New obstetric maneuver for dystocia. JAMA 1954; 155:1442.
57. Maughan GB. The safe and simple delivery of persistent posterior and transverse positions. Am J Obstet Gynecol 1956; 71:741–745.
58. Magnin P, Andra P. Est-il legitime de faire aujourd-hui des grandes rotations au forceps? Rev Fr Gynecol Obstet 1984; 79:255–261.
59. Seides S. A "two forceps maneuver" for persistent occipitoposterior presentation. Surg Gynecol Obstet 1923; 36:421–426.
60. Posner AC, Friedman S, Posner LB. Modern trends in the management of face and brow presentations. Surg Gynecol Obstet 1957; 104:485–490.
61. Posner LB, Rubin EJ, Posner AC. Face and brow presentations: a continuing study. Obstet Gynecol 1963; 21:745–749, .
62. Rudolph SJ. Face presentation. Am J Obstet Gynecol 1947; 54:987–993.
63. Moore EJT, Dennen EH. Management of persistent brow presentation. Obstet Gynecol 1955; 6:186–189.
64. Reddoch JW. Face presentation. Am J Obstet Gynecol 1948; 56:86–99.
65. Gomez HE, Dennen EH. Face presentation: a study of 45 consecutive cases. Obstet Gynecol 1956; 8:103–106.
66. Hellman LM, Apperson JWW, Connally F. Face and brow presentation. Am J Obstet Gynecol 1950; 59:831–842.

4

Vacuum Extraction Operations

I believe that the construction of the air tractor is still very far from being so perfect as it will yet be rendered.

JR SIMPSON, 1849 (1)

We much fear that this proposed substitute for forceps may only lead to disappointment. We almost dread the infant's scalp being torn off or a parietal bone dragged out. Our fears may be visionary and certainly the communication of Professor Simpson is most deserving of attention. Before approving of the proposal, we must wait to see it fully tested and practiced.

Editorial, *London Journal of Medicine* I, 283, 1849

Applications

Introduction

Modern vacuum extractors consist of a metal or plastic cup connected by a flexible silastic or rubber tubing to a vacuum source. Properly engineered devices include a vacuum trap between the cup and vacuum source, both to protect the vacuum mechanism as well as to provide a visual check on the volume and character of any aspirated material. The system also includes a vacuum pump which varies the strength of the suction, a gauge to measure the negative pressure produced, and usually a separate hand and/or foot valve to permit the operator to rapidly interrupt the suction. Vacuum for delivery can be produced in a number of ways. A specialized pump for the vacuum extractor can be used (Medela Corp., Crystal Lake, IL; Egnell/Ameda, Inc., Cary, IL), a hand pump (Columbia Medical and Surgical, Inc., Lake Oswego, OR), or even wall suction, as long as the strength of the vacuum can be measured and controlled. Modern extractor pumps are best, as they automatically maintain a preset pressure, compensating for the inevitable imperfection of the seal and minute leaks elsewhere in the system.

Forces in Vacuum Extraction

The purpose of the vacuum extractor is to create a tractive force on the fetal scalp to assist the normal forces of labor (2–6). In using these devices, negative pressure holds the vacuum cup in apposition to the fetal scalp (Fig. 4.1). Dependent upon the type of device and the length of application, a characteristic mound of edema and hemorrhagic fluid accumulates in the subcutaneous tissues of the scalp as a result of the localized vacuum. Thus, an artificial caput succedaneum, termed the *chignon*, is produced (Fig. 4.2). Chignon is the French word for a large coil or hump of hair drawn into a bun at the back of the head. This artificial caput succedaneum does not differ from the spontaneous caput succedaneum except in etiology. "Nor-

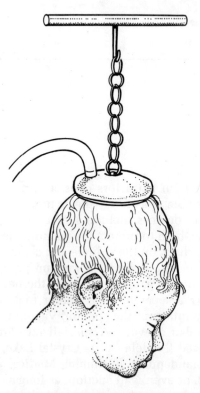

Figure 4.1. Correct midoccipital application of rigid-cup vacuum extractor (Bird's modification).

mal" caput is produced when uterine contractions force the fetal head against an undilated cervix resulting in differential pressure against the fetal scalp, with resultant edema formation (7). In most instances the chignon is of cosmetic concern only and rapidly resolves postpartum.

The tractive force applied by the operator to the cup is transmitted to the fetal scalp through the traction handle. Thiery (6) likens the process of scalp traction to a ball (the fetal head) pulled along in a string bag (the scalp). As tension is applied to the scalp the fetal head is partially compressed. The force applied is transmitted to the attachment of the scalp at the circumference of the fetal skull, theoretically producing relatively limited compression of the cranium, at least in comparison to certain forceps applications (6). With the classic Malmström instrument the maximum force possible is approximately 13–14 kg but can exceed 20 kg with a firm application or elevated pressure (6, 8). For comparison, during spontaneous labor the maximal expulsive force acting on the fetal head approximates 15 kg (9). Greater force leads to disengagement of the cup or sustained vacuum leakage. This spontaneous cup displacement is considered a safety factor by proponents of vacuum extraction (10). For example, Saling and Hartung (8) observed that the Malmström cup was detached from the fetal scalp in 10/22 (45%) deliveries if the tractive force met or exceeded 20 kg. However, if the force applied was less than 20 kg, no detachments oc-

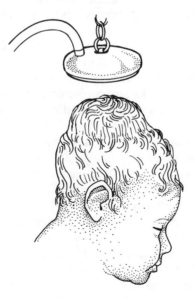

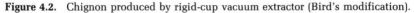

Figure 4.2.   Chignon produced by rigid-cup vacuum extractor (Bird's modification).

curred. When compared to the Malmström-type vacuum extractor, classic obstetrical forceps generate substantially greater forces in similar clinical circumstances although, as will be reviewed, all data on cranial forces in vacuum extraction and comparable forceps deliveries are highly controversial and subject to considerable variation (11).

Pressure changes both on and within the fetal head have been studied for forceps- and vacuum-assisted delivery, both in clinical settings as well as in the laboratory, with no uniformity of opinion as to results (11, 12–14, 18, 19). However, some useful conclusions can fairly be drawn from these data. Vacuum cup displacement depends upon the strength of the vacuum, height of the cup, as well as the angle of traction (6). Using a series of mathematic models, Rosa calculated that the maximum tractive force for the vacuum extractor, that is, the force applied before a 55-mm Malmström-type cup evacuated to 0.5 kg/cm^2 will break loose, amounts to 14.8 kg. In general, clinical studies support this contention. Further, Rosa noted that, if the plane of traction was not perpendicular to the surface of the cup, the maximal tractive force obtainable decreased in proportion to the obliquity of the angle (12). Angular pulls reduced the net-effective force obtainable with the extractor due to lifting of the cup edge and loss of vacuum. Put more simply, cup dislodgment occurred at progressively lower vacuum pressures as the pull became increasingly oblique. Rosa estimated that the intracranial pressure produced by the average pull of 10 kg amounted to 75 g/cm^2. He further estimated that with a pull of the same magnitude applied by forceps, the compressible force between the tips of the instrument was some 20 times greater (1400 g/cm^2) and even higher between the blades (6). In support of Rosa's calculations, data on *in vitro* measurement of tractive forces and head compression suggest less fetal head compression with the vacuum extractor than with forceps. For example, Roman and Dinca (15) directly measured intracranial pressures in studies on dead newborns. An increase of 1–2 mm Hg (torr) was recorded with a vacuum extractor. When forceps were applied, marked increases of 18–25 torr and occasional pressure increases as high as 35 torr were observed. Roman calculated that forceps application was associated with a 15–20-fold greater increase in cranial compressive force than could be produced by a equally vigorous vacuum extraction (15). However, there is not a uniformity of opinion on these points. According to Moolgaoker et al. (13), during spontaneous vaginal delivery average cranial compression varies from 1.9 to 2.9 psi, dependent upon maternal parity and station of the fetal head. By their measurements cranial pressure was 4.6 psi during vacuum extraction and 3.0–4.4 psi with instrumental delivery for a variety of forceps models. These differences became greater when the total compressive force produced by the two types of instruments were compared. In the report of Moolgaoker and colleagues, the apparent disadvantage of the vacuum extractor occurred largely because vacuum delivery required more time for delivery than forceps. However, data from clinical studies is contradictory (16). For example, in the Portsmouth operative delivery trial in which 304 women were randomly assigned to vacuum extraction or forceps delivery, both the mean length of the second stage and the interval between random assignment of instrument and delivery was the same (17). Thus, not surprisingly technique and experience figure in the amount of force generated during a specific parturition. It appears that the vacuum extractor *can* generate cranial pressures similar to forceps but that this is the exception rather than the rule as long as the recommendations for application are closely followed.

Clinical Use

Success in vacuum extraction is due to careful choice of cases, close attention to detail, and an understanding of the mechanism of labor. Successful accouchement by vacuum extraction is dependent upon the judicious application of force, recruitment of maternal assistance in expulsive efforts, and a proper relationship between fetal and maternal size (Table 4.1).

If the rigid Malmström cup is chosen, the *largest* practical size should be used. Normally, only the 50-mm cup is in use on our service. In general, the greater the cup diameter, the greater the tractive force possible, and the less likely is cup detachment.

Ideally, the vacuum apparatus used should automatically maintain constant negative pressure as set by a control valve. Complete or partial loss of vacuum permits cup detachment with loss of traction and possible scalp injury. Alternatively, if the vacuum applied is excessive, while greater force can be applied before loss of the cup adhesion, fetal scalp injury is more likely. Normally, the working vacuum for vacuum extractors is 0.8 kg/cm^2 (550–600 torr). Use of greater

Table 4.1.   Factors Influencing Effective Vacuum Extraction[a]

Cup design: shape, size, and traction site attachment
Consistency and strength of vacuum
Maternal cervical dilatation
Strength of maternal expulsive efforts and coordination with traction
Fetal size and the extent of cephalopelvic disproportion
Station and deflection of the fetal head
Angle and technique of traction

[a]Modified from Thiery M. Obstetric vacuum extraction. Obstet Gynecol Annu 1985; 14:73–111.

vacuums increases the traction force possible with a given extractor but also rapidly increases the likelihood of fetal injury (19).

As reviewed under "Indications for Vacuum Extraction" and "Contraindications to Vacuum Extraction," the author does not favor use of vacuum extraction if the cervix is undilated except in unusual instances of fetal distress and only while preparations for cesarean delivery are under way, despite there being considerable European literature supporting such applications. The exception is in instances of fetal distress in multiparas at 7 cm or greater when cephalopelvic disproportion is not an issue. If application of the vacuum extractor is restricted to patients with full dilatation, cervical dystocia cannot be a factor obstructing or slowing descent.

The same considerations of fetopelvic disproportion govern vacuum extraction and forceps. The larger the fetus, the more difficult the pull and the greater likelihood of either failure, scalp injury, or shoulder girdle dystocia. Particular care is necessary in trials of vaginal delivery when the outcome of extraction is uncertain and fetal size difficult to estimate.

The station and deflection of the fetal head are important in correct vacuum extraction application and traction (18, 20). If the fetal head extends or rotates laterally due to improper cup placement, a progressively larger cranial diameter is presented to the birth canal, compounding the problem of cephalopelvic disproportion. Regardless of type, the vacuum cup should always be located in the midline toward the fetal occiput (Fig. 4.3A). In this location, the head will be flexed and not extended when traction is applied. Too anterior an application tends to deflex the fetal head (Fig. 4.3C) presenting a larger diameter to the birth canal. Oblique applications are equally bad, as they tend to accentuate cranial asynclitism as traction is applied (Fig. 4.3B). This point is not sufficiently emphasized in most descriptions of vacuum extraction. Failure to correctly position the cup to favor cranial flexion is likely the greatest factor in failure of extraction from the midpelvis. If the Malmström cup has been chosen, the "OP" model (Bird's modification) should be used for cases of persisting occiput posterior positions or transverse arrests with accompanying deflection/asynclitism.

The vacuum extractor, regardless of design, must be accorded the same respect as forceps. Prior to any attempted extraction, careful attention is given to alternative management, including oxytocin ad-

Table 4.2. The Three Checks for Correct Application of the Vacuum Extractor

No maternal tissue included under cup margin
Cup covers the fetal occiput, in the midline
Marker or vacuum port of suction cup points toward the occiput

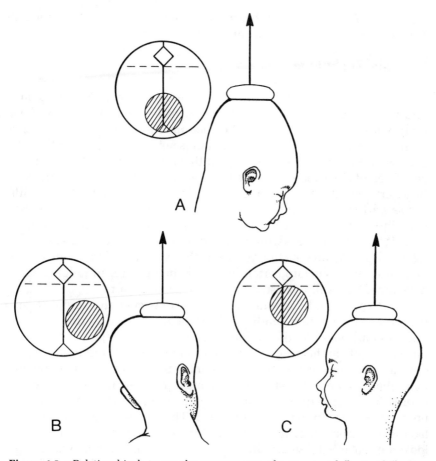

Figure 4.3. Relationship between the vacuum cup placement and flexion/deflection and asynclitism of the fetal head. A rigid metal (Malmström) cup is depicted. However, these principles of placement are valid for all types of vacuum extractors (see text for details). (Modified from Bird GC. The use of the vacuum extractor. Clin Obstet Gynaecol 1982; 9:641–661.

ministration, continued observation, forceps application, and/or cesarean section. Once vacuum extraction has been chosen and the instrument applied, "checks" similar to those used with forceps are performed by the operator (Table 4.2). The importance of an occipital application has already been emphasized. Maternal tissue must be excluded from the cup to avoid both a poor seal and maternal injury. Finally, alignment of a marker or the vacuum port toward the occiput permits observation of rotation as the presenting part descends.

During the application of negative pressure, fetal bradycardias can occur (20). The release of vacuum between contractions results in a prompt return of the fetal heart rate to normal and helps distinguish this iatrogenic bradycardia from true fetal distress.

Traction Technique

In traction, a two-handed technique is used. The index and middle fingers of the nontraction hand make contact with the fetal scalp while the thumb pushes the vacuum cup against the fetal head with backward pressure during traction (see illustration under "Applications" (16). Malmström argues that this *Dreifingergriff* ("three-finger grip") results in a vector of force that follows the pelvic curve. Further, he asserts that during spontaneous vaginal delivery the fetal head fails to use part of the "hind pelvis," and that, using this counterpressure technique with each pull, this extra posterior space can be utilized (16). Whether these assertions are true or not, counterpressure may retard cup detachment. In any event, the presence of the nontraction hand thumb on the cup certainly assists the operator in judging early detachment as well as descent of the presenting part.

Experienced vacuum extractor accoucheurs are careful to apply force to the traction handle *at the same time* as the uterine contraction. If at all possible, the patient is encouraged to augment these expulsive efforts by bearing down at the same time. Maternal efforts coordinated to uterine contractions are most important, as the extractor, more than forceps, is designed to *augment* and not simply replace the natural forces of delivery. In vacuum extraction, as in forceps delivery, progress is more important than speed. The vacuum cup tends to detach if the direction of traction deviates from the optimal; this can be looked upon as a safeguard. In fact, the major cause of cup detachment is failure to pull perpendicular to the plane of the cup through the pelvic curve (Carus' curve). Depending upon the station of the fetal head, the operator may need to sit, have the delivery table elevated, or in unusual circumstances even kneel to reach the correct angle of pull.

Vacuum extraction can be expected to fail in 1–3% of cases (10). Uncommonly, if vacuum extraction fails, forceps can be applied and delivery achieved safely. In the author's experience, this is usually when the vacuum extractor has been incorrectly applied or mechanical correction of deflection or rotation of the fetal head is needed before progress can occur. Such clinical circumstances are uncommon and in this setting maternal injuries are more frequent (22). *If during an attempted delivery the vacuum extractor has become detached twice or no station is made during traction, the greatest of care must be exercised before forceps are applied or vacuum extraction attempted again.* There is reason for caution. More difficult cases of dystocia involve enhanced maternal and fetal risks. It is no surprise that when forceps are used following failure of vacuum extraction, vaginal lacerations are common (22). For example, Greis (23) observed increased fetal compromise when forceps were used following a failed vacuum extraction. Maternal risks in such a setting are not inconsequential either.

Lasbrey and coworkers (24) reported on 233 cases of vacuum extraction. In 77% of their cases, delivery occurred after one to five pulls, with an incident of cerebral trauma of 1.2%. In the remaining cases, if six or more pulls were necessary, cerebral trauma was observed in 11%. Sjöstedt's data on nearly 1500 attempted instrumental deliveries are helpful (Table 4.3) (3). Approximately 90% of the nearly 1500 instrumental deliveries he studied were completed with four tractions or less. The message from these data is clear. *The vast majority of vacuum extractions (and forceps deliveries) are rapidly and easily accomplished. If attempted delivery does not begin with the first traction, it should be abandoned.* Heroics have no place in instrumental vaginal delivery.

In sum, the best rule is to permit no more than five tractions with uterine contractions or two episodes of breaking of suction in any trial of vacuum extraction (Table 4.3). *Further, if no station is made beginning with the first traction effort,* the vacuum extraction should be considered to have failed and an alternative form of delivery initiated. If vacuum extraction fails and the decision is made to move to cesarean delivery, an assistant should be placed under the operative drapes to displace the fetal head upward by vaginal manipulation to avoid injury to the lower uterine segment during extraction.

Coding of Applications

Traditionally vacuum extractor procedures have not been reported in a similar fashion as forceps operations, although there are

Table 4.3. Number of Tractions Required to Achieve Delivery in 1497 Cases of Assisted Vacuum Extraction and Forceps Delivery[a]

No. of Traction Efforts	Malmström Vacuum Extractor (N = 433)	Forceps (N = 555)
1–2	296 (68.4%)	213 (38.4%)
3–4	108 (24.9%)	270 (48.6%)
≥5	29 (6.7%)	72 (12.9%)

[a]Neonates <600 g excluded; other exclusions include breech presentations, cesarean section deliveries, transverse lies, and multiple gestations. Twins were included if >600 g and one delivered spontaneously, by vertex. Modified from Sjöstedt JE. The vacuum extractor and forceps in obstetrics: A clinical study. Acta Obstet Gynecol Scand 1967; 46 (suppl 10):3–208.

cogent reasons for similar coding. Part of the difficulty surrounds the questions of rotation. This is where forceps applications and vacuum procedures diverse sharply. True midpelvic forceps procedures with rotation of more than 45° clearly increase maternal/fetal risk of injury and this is reflected in the American College of Obstetricians and Gynecologists (ACOG) coding descriptions (Table 2.1). As the vacuum extractor does not *impose* rotation in the same fashion as forceps, these coding criteria lack the same implications when the ventouse is applied. For the purposes of this discussion, vacuum operations will be described as *mid, low* or *outlet* procedures, using the same criteria of *station* as the parallel forceps operations without, however, consideration of rotation.

Malpresentation and Rotation

Management of occipitoposterior and occipitolateral positions of the fetal head are controversial, whether by vacuum extraction or forceps (see Chapter 3). In the course of labor, approximately 10% of such presentations will require assistance. A number of possible management methods have been suggested: forceps rotation by Kielland forceps, the Scanzoni maneuver, vacuum extraction, manual rotation followed by forceps or vacuum or cesarean section. With either manual or forceps rotation, the level of the rotation and direction are imposed by the operator. A possible advantage of the vacuum extractor is that the head is free to rotate in the most favorable direction, depending upon the head shape and the anatomy of the pelvis as labor progresses (22). It may be that this fact gives the fetal head a better chance of adapting to pelvic architecture. It is countered that in circumstances of abnormalities of pelvic anatomy a trained accoucheur may be better able to manipulate the head through the pelvis when the "natural" processes have failed. Chalmers (2) described a series of 2300 occipitoposterior cases delivered at Wooster Royal Infirmary; 261 or 11.3% required assisted delivery with the vacuum extractor. In 65 cases, with traction, the fetus rotated to an occiput anterior position. That author reported no "undue" maternal trauma, no perinatal mortality, and little morbidity. In a retrospective series of 256 vacuum extractions compared to 300 forceps deliveries, Broekhuizen and coworkers (22) noted that autorotation from occiput posterior/transverse to an anterior position occurred in 88/152 instances (58%), comparable to the active rotation required in 43/81 or 53% of posterior/transverse cases managed by forceps application.

Avoidance of Fetal Injury

Lesions of the scalp are the invariable result of vacuum extraction (2, 22, 24, 25). The majority of these are minor and resolve spontaneously; however, significant trauma is not uncommon, especially if the operator is inexperienced (26, 27). Reduction in the incidence of scalp trauma is dependent upon careful selection of cases, rigorous attention to limitations of the period of traction, and close adherence to the two-handed technique of traction with avoidance of cup detachment, particularly "popping off" of the cup (Table 4.4). Scalp lesions are particularly likely when care is not given to early signs of cup detachment during traction. These include lifting of the cup edge and hearing a sucking noise as the suction begins to fail. Too rapid induction of vacuum, failure to await caput succedaneum formation if the rigid vacuum extractor is used, continuous traction in the absence of uterine contractions, prolonged application of the extractor, and use of excessive vacuum also contribute to scalp injury.

Bird (20) strongly cautions against what he terms "negative traction." Negative traction is defined as traction insufficient to cause the fetal head to descend in the birth canal, but not strong enough to detach the suction cup. This is particularly dangerous, as it causes the scalp to descend without the skull, pulling the galea away from the cranium. This may rupture the emissary veins, resulting in bleeding into the loose subgaleal tissue. Without providing data, Bird argues that grossly edematous scalps are more easily injured and that bald scalps are more prone to abrasion than those with abundant hair. In general, extraction of premature infants is to be avoided (28).

Vacuum extraction fails for several reasons (Table 4.5). The cup can fail to accept strong traction due to the presence of a large caput succedaneum, oblique traction, leaks or faults in the apparatus, or entrapment in the cup of maternal or fetal tissue. If the cup does accept strong traction yet descent does not occur, cephalopelvic disproportion, an application producing cranial extension rather than

Table 4.4. Rules for Clinical Use of Vacuum Extractors

Traction is bimanual in the pelvic curve with close attention to cup detachment and *Dreifingergriff*
All applications are subject to "three checks" prior to traction
Traction augments spontaneous or induced uterine contractions
Maximum time for cup application is 25 minutes
Maximum of five traction pulls
Maximum of two cup detachments
Advancement of fetal head should begin with the *first* attempted traction
Applications to premature infants (<37 weeks) are to be avoided

Table 4.5.   Causes of Vacuum Extraction Failure

Fetopelvic disproportion
  Fetal macrosomia
  Pelvic inadequacy or malformation
Dystocia
  Fetal or maternal tumor
  Conjoined or locking twins
  High presenting part
  Undilated cervix
  Deflexed or posterior position of fetal head
Technical errors
  Vacuum leakage
  Incomplete or defective equipment
  Failure to allow for chignon formation when using rigid cups
  Oblique traction leading to cup detachment
  Failure to apply traction smoothly, using Dreifingergriff

flexion, or pulling in the wrong direction—i.e., not in the correct pelvic curve—are likely explanations.

Vacuum Extraction Instruments

The most common instruments in use in the United States for vacuum extraction are the flexible Kobayashi-design silastic instrument and Bird's modification of the Malmström cup. The disposable plastic cup (Mityvac) is also available and has achieved a unique popularity in out-of-hospital accouchements.

Flexible Vacuum Extractor (Kobayashi Device)

This instrument (silastic obstetrical vacuum cup, Dow Corning Corp., Midland, MI) consists of an obstetric vacuum cup, a 208-mm-long device, constructed of soft, translucent, silicone elastimer (29) (Fig. 4.4). The end is flared into a cone- or cup-shaped segment, 65 mm in diameter. A blue marking or indicator line is incorporated into the plastic of the cup. There are three ridges molded into the shaft, serving as potential traction sites for the operator. Fitted in the handle are a chrome-plated brass grip with a plunger-actuated valve mechanism to release the vacuum. A presumed advantage of Kobayashi's design is that the cup is soft, permitting easier vaginal insertion and automatic adjustment to the fetal head. Further, due to the flexibility of the device, the waiting period for the development of a working vacuum is minimal, and slow incremental increases in vacuum to produce the classic chignon is not required. As the cup is designed to mold itself over the fetal occiput, likelihood of scalp injury is theoretically reduced (30–35). A disadvantage of this device is its tendency to fail more frequently than the Malmström cup, particularly in occiput pos-

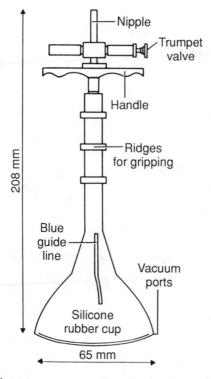

208 mm

65 mm

Nipple

Trumpet valve

Handle

Ridges for gripping

Blue guide line

Vacuum ports

Silicone rubber cup

Figure 4.4.   Silastic obstetric vacuum cup (Dow Corning Corp.). (Reprinted from Witter FR. Soft-cup vacuum extractors safely assist normal deliveries. Contemp Obstet Gynecol 1985; 26(suppl):109–119.

terior positions (35). The extractor darkens considerably with age and the cumulative effects of multiple sterilizations but these changes in appearance do not appear to adversely affect performance (19).

Rigid Metal Cup Vacuum Extractor (Malmström and Bird's Modified Device)

The most common metal cup extractor in the armamentarium of most obstetrical services is Bird's modification of the original Malmström design (Fig. 4.5) (36). Cups are produced in varying sizes; however, those of 50 mm are most useful. The device is made of stainless steel with a rolled, smooth edge. The lateral vacuum port within the cup is protected by a plastic mesh. Traction is applied by a detachable handle that hooks to a centrally fixed chain.

The only technical problems we have encountered with the Bird cup is inadvertent dislodgment of the vacuum tubing during vaginal insertion or dropping of the unsecured traction handle during as-

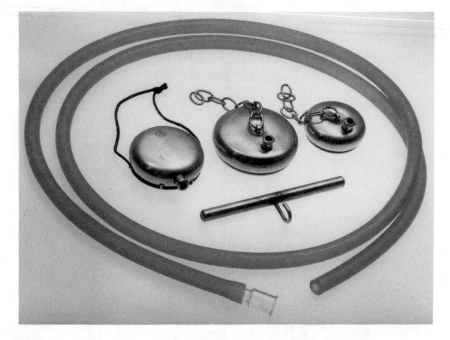

Figure 4.5. Bird's modification of Malmström vacuum extractor cup (36). Note eccentrically located vacuum port and the separate, permanently affixed traction chain. Cup with the lateral port and nylon cord is the "OP" model for deflexed or occiput posterior positions.

sembly of the device or when vaginal examinations are performed between traction pulls. The tubing is most difficult to insert correctly once the cup is in apposition to the fetal scalp. If inadvertent disconnection occurs, it is necessary to remove the cup from the birth canal, refit the tubing over the suction port, and repeat the application. On occasion, a ligature is used to secure the vacuum tubing to the suction port. On our service, the traction handle has been so frequently dropped on the floor that we fabricated additional handles with an exaggerated curve in the traction hook to reduce the possibility of disarticulation. It is prudent to keep a spare handle separately wrapped and sterilized to offset this eventuality, especially in a teaching setting.

Plastic Disposable Vacuum Extractor (Mityvac Vacuum Extraction Delivery System)

This unique device (Mityvac Vacuum Extraction Delivery System, Columbia Medical and Surgical, Inc., Lake Oswego, OR) consists of a one-piece molded polyethylene 60-mm plastic cup with attached handle (37, 38) (Fig. 4.6). The cup border is flared and semirigid and comes in one size only. As the device is all one piece, assembly is not

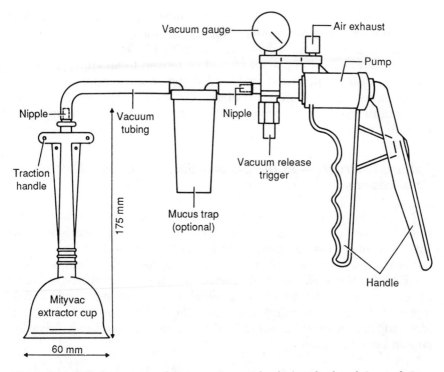

Figure 4.6. Mityvac vacuum delivery system (Columbia Medical and Surgical, Inc., Lake Oswego, OR). The device is molded from flexible plastic and designed to be disposable. (Reprinted from Witter FR. Soft-cup vacuum extractors safely assist normal deliveries. Contemp Obstet Gynecol 1985; 26(suppl):109–119.

required. It is supplied presterilized and is designed to be disposable. A plastic, nondisposable hand vacuum pump is available as part of this extraction system but the cup will operate on any vacuum system.

Indications for Vacuum Extraction

Failure to Progress in the Second Stage of Labor: Indicated Applications

Inability to expel the fetus in the second stage of labor is the classic indication for instrumental delivery. When progress ceases, the clinician must assess the fetal and maternal condition with particular attention to malposition (occiput posterior (OP), deflexed head) and fetal macrosomia. As long as the fetal heart rate tracing is acceptable, maternal exhaustion is not present, and some progress is being made, the accoucheur may delay intervention. Thus the older, rigid "2-hour" second stage rule is no longer considered valid. Once the decision is made to intervene, the patient should be moved to an appropriate locale, the instrument introduced, and delivery accomplished. Any of the vacuum extractors may be chosen. Following occipital placement and careful checking of the application, traction is produced and parturition follows.

Failure to Progress in the Second Stage of Labor: Elective Applications

In theory, the vacuum extractor can be used as an outlet instrument to assist final expulsion of the fetal head. Such applications have little advantage over forceps, if any. The author prefers forceps for outlet delivery, as they are rapid, easy, and generally atraumatic in such applications. However, if anesthesia is limited or absent, a flexible or semirigid extractor can be applied in the usual manner to assist delivery. In outlet applications either the Mityvac extractor or the Malmström instrument are less likely to dislodge than the Kobayashi cup and are preferred.

Extraction of the Second Twin

The vacuum extractor is quite effective in assisting at twin delivery. If the parturient meets the criteria for a trial of labor with twins, a vacuum extractor and forceps are prepared for possible use (38). Following delivery—either assisted or spontaneous—of the first or leading twin, the position of the second is promptly confirmed by vaginal examination and real time ultrasound scanning. With bimanual assistance the cephalic pole is positioned over the pelvis and the membranes ruptured. Oxytocin may then be administered or the accoucheur may simply wait. Real time ultrasound observes the fetal heart rate during these manipulations. The vacuum extractor is introduced and pressed gently against the oncoming fetal head. Prompt production of negative pressure grasps the fetal head without loss of station. After careful check of application, traction is produced with uterine contractions, usually achieving delivery rapidly. There are no major contraindications to this procedure except marked fetal prematurity. The operator must use care to avoid displacing the fetal head out of the pelvis, be certain of the occipital placement of the vacuum cup, and avoid trapping maternal or fetal tissues under the cup edge.

Trial of Vaginal Delivery

The vacuum extractor is the instrument of choice in circumstances where fetal distress is not present and a *trial* of midpelvic extraction is contemplated. As such circumstances are frequently accompanied by a heavily molded head and/or caput succedaneum, the vacuum extractor is particularly well-suited to such trials, as its application is easier than forceps, less likely to displace the fetal head to a higher station, and does not increase the diameter of the mass to be extracted. The operator needs to be acutely aware of the characteristics of a *trial*. (see Chapter 2, "Trial versus Failed Forceps"). A trial is just that, attempted delivery with preparation (equipment, personnel, etc.) for cesarean delivery if the attempted accouchement fails. Further, the practitioner must approach the application with a clear plan of attack. Some practitioners will utilize the vacuum extractor to make station, with the intention of removing the device and replacing it with forceps once it is apparent that descent is possible. Other accoucheurs will simply conduct the entire extraction with the originally applied instrument.

Extraction at Cesarean Section

A number of clinicians have used the vacuum extractor to assist in cesarean delivery (Table 4.6). The flexible or semirigid cups are best for this application. A thin lower uterine segment in a woman with a narrow pelvis predisposes to laceration when manual extraction of the fetal head is performed. In such circumstances, the head can be grasped with the ventouse and the infant promptly extracted without trauma to mother or infant.

Fetal Distress or Poor Progress in the First Stage of Labor

European authorities such as Chamberlain (44) state that "indications for vacuum extractions are found mostly in the first stage of labour. . . ." He describes the use of vacuum extraction for fetal distress in multiparous patients at or beyond 7 cm of dilatation. Other authors have reported successful use of vacuum extraction for fetal distress, even with cord prolapse (45–47). In the absence of fetal distress, application of the vacuum extractor through an undilated cervix and with traction with each contraction has been claimed to result in prompt, complete dilatation and delivery (5, 6, 44, 48). In American practice, fetal distress before complete cervical dilatation is usually managed by cesarean delivery.

Table 4.6. Vacuum-assisted Delivery at Cesarean Section

Author	Successful Cases	Instrument	Comments
Solomons (40)		Malmström cup	No complications reported
Bercovici (41)	20/22 (91%)	Malmström cup	Small caput succedaneum in "all infants," 5/20 (25%) infants experienced mild increases in bilirubin
Pelosi & Apuzzio (42)	35/35 (100%)	Silastic cup[a]	12/35 (34%) infants experienced "minimal" caput succedaneum
Boehm (43)	50/50 (100%)	Silastic cup[a]	No complications reported

[a]Silastic obstetrical vacuum cup (Medical Products, Dow Corning Corp.).

Fetal Distress in the Second Stage of Labor

The vacuum extractor can be used to assist delivery in fully dilated patients when disproportion is not a clinical question, a reasonable station of the fetal head exists, and evidence of fetal distress is present. Forceps are likely a better choice in this setting for many clinicians, unless one is well-trained in the vacuum extraction technique and the apparatus can be promptly assembled and applied. It is best to position the patient for prompt vaginal delivery while making simultaneous preparations for cesarean section in case vaginal instrumental delivery fails.

Contraindications to Vacuum Extraction

Contraindications to vacuum extraction are in general similar to those for forceps application (Table 4.7). In abnormal presentations, such as face or breech, the extractor should not be applied due to the possibility of fetal injury and the technical problem of achieving an adequate seal. With care, the vacuum extractor can safely be applied to the fetal head at higher station than possible with forceps. However, the question is not whether the vacuum extractor can be applied at high station but why it is clinically indicated or desirable to do so. There are very few clinical settings, except perhaps delivery of second twins, and rarely in fetal distress, when such applications are appropriate.

Prior scalp sampling is sometimes cited as a contraindication to the use of the vacuum extractor (49). However, Thiery (50) observed no instances of neonatal exsanguination among more than 1000 vacuum extractions involving neonates who had been monitored with an electrode attached to the fetal scalp from which a blood sample had been taken at full dilatation.

Table 4.7. Contraindications to Vacuum Extraction[a]

Absolute
  Face presentation
  Breech presentation
  True cephalopelvic disproportion (CPD)
  High head[b]
Relative
  Fetal distress
  Undilated cervix
  Fetal demise
  Congenital abnormalities of cranium
  Premature infants (<37 weeks)[b]

[a]From Halme J, Ekbladh L. The vacuum extractor for obstetric delivery. Clin Obstet Gynaecol 1982; 25:167–175.
[b]A partial exception exists for second twins (see text).

If the fetus is dead and particularly if a rigid metal extractor is used, failure is common, as a chignon will not form normally. If fetal demise occurred long enough in advance to delivery such that maceration is advanced, the cranium is usually not a barrier to delivery due to its extreme flaccidity. If assisted delivery is required, forceps are a better choice.

While European literature prominently mentions fetal distress as an indication for vacuum extraction, practice in the United States is inherently more conservative and dependent largely upon cesarean section or forceps delivery if *in utero* distress is diagnosed. This is largely due to inexperience with vacuum extraction and the belief—in many instances valid—that vacuum extraction takes longer to deliver an infant than does forceps, due to the need to assemble the instrument, attach vacuum, etc. Part of this concern is perhaps invalid as the Portsmouth study indicates, that, *on average in experienced hands,* vacuum extraction is equally rapid as forceps in achieving delivery (17).

The use of vacuum extraction in the delivery of preterm infants, except second twins, is not advised, due largely to concern over intracranial injury although some authors indicate no unusual complications from such applications (28). Second twins are a partial exception, as their delivery requires minimal tractive force because of prior cervical and vaginal dilatation with the passage of the first infant (39).

Technique: Outlet Vacuum Extraction

Definition

Outlet vacuum extraction is the cephalic application of the vacuum extractor at full cervical dilatation when the fetal skull has reached the pelvic floor, the fetal head is at or in the perineum, and the scalp is visible at the introitus without spreading the labia, regardless of position.

Prerequisites

(a) Appropriate occipital, midline application of vacuum cup;
(b) Analgesia (if required)
  • Pudendal nerve block,
  • Saddle block,
  • (Uncommonly) epidural anesthesia,
  • (Rarely) general anesthesia;
(c) Operator certainty of fetal station and position. Pelvic examination to establish the station, position, and deflection of the fetal head;
(d) Empty maternal bladder (Credé, recent voiding);
(e) Full cervical dilatation;
(f) Ruptured membranes.

Application

1. With the patient prepared for delivery and adequate analgesia present, a pelvic examination reconfirms the fetal position, station, and deflection of the fetal head. The cup is then ghosted against the perineum prior to attempting an application (Fig. 4.7). Note in the accompanying illustration that the vacuum port of Bird's modification of the Malmström cup is aligned pointing toward the posterior fontanelle of the fetal head. If the silastic cup is used, the inscribed blue line should be oriented in the same fashion. With the Mityvac instrument, one handle may be so directed. This provides a marker for the clinician to follow during descent and/or rotation of the presenting part. This maneuver exactly parallels ghosting of forceps prior to application and should not be omitted, as it orients the operator and forces rethinking of the entire operation.

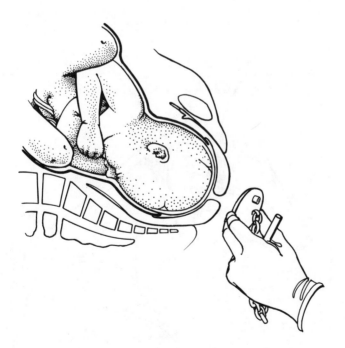

Figure 4.7. OA position: outlet extraction. Ghosting the metal cup vacuum extractor (Bird's modification) prior to attempting application. Note that the vacuum hose has not been attached in this illustration.

2. The cup is lubricated with surgical soap or gel and turned sideways and gently pressed through the labia into the vaginal canal as the perineal body is depressed by the operator's finger (Fig. 4.8). Note that the vacuum tubing is attached *prior* to attempting insertion of the vacuum cup.

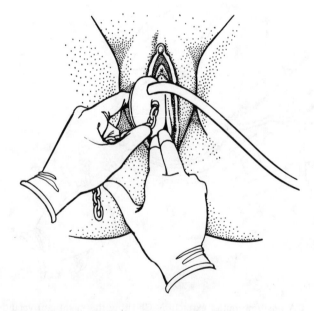

Figure 4.8. Outlet vacuum extraction. Inserting metal cup vacuum extractor (Bird's modification) through the labia.

3. The operator then presses the cup gently against the fetal head, orienting it over the center of the posterior fontanelle. The operator then sweeps his/her finger around the cup to be certain no maternal tissues are entrapped (Fig. 4.9). When certain that the cup margins are clear, a light vacuum is produced to initially seal the cup to the fetal head. The application is then carefully rechecked before full vacuum is applied or traction is attempted.

Checks for the vacuum extractor, regardless of type:

(a) No maternal tissue included under the cup margin;
(b) Cup covers the fetal occiput, in the midline;
(c) Marker or handle (soft cup instruments) or vacuum port (Malmström instrument) points toward the fetal occiput.

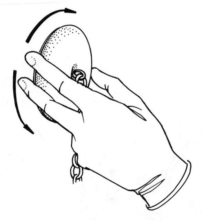

Figure 4.9.   Vacuum extraction. Correct application of vacuum cup is verified.

4. Once certain that the application is accurate, the operator increases the pressure by 0.2 kg/cm^2 at intervals of 1–2 minutes, producing the chignon. Full operative pressure is 0.8 kg/cm^2 (550–600 torr). With the silastic instrument, formation of the chignon is not required and full operative vacuum may be applied at once with traction immediately following.

5. *Traction is now applied in the pelvic curve in a similar fashion to a forceps operation* (Fig. 4.10). An episiotomy is performed, as necessary. Tension on the extractor handle is allowed to build gradually, paralleling the uterine contractions. Between contractions, tension is released and the vacuum is maintained at the discretion of the surgeon. During tractive efforts the operator places two fingers of the *nontraction* hand on the fetal scalp with his/her thumb on the cup edge (*Dreifingergriff*). Counter traction *against* the cup is applied with the operator's thumb. With this technique, descent of the presenting part and lifting or early separation of the cup is palpable. Thus, rapid detachment or popping off of the cup is less likely. A similar bimanual technique is used with all types of vacuum extractors. Descent should occur *with the first traction.* Failure to make station immediately requires prompt reassessment.

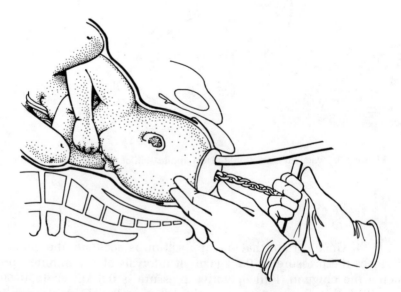

Figure 4.10.   OA position. Outlet vacuum extraction. *Dreifingergriff* (three-finger grip) traction with metal cup vacuum extractor (Bird's modification).

6. When the fetal head crowns, suction is interrupted and the vacuum cup detached after the fetal chin is grasped by Ritgen's maneuver (Fig. 4.11). Delivery of the body follows in the usual fashion.

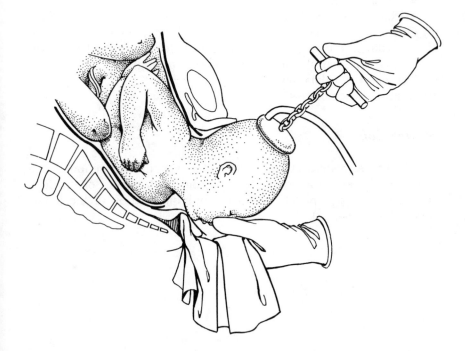

Figure 4.11. OA position. Vacuum extraction. Delivery and Ritgen's maneuver with metal cup vacuum extractor (Bird's modification).

Technique: Low and Midpelvic Extraction

Definition

Low vacuum extraction is the cephalic application of the vacuum extractor at full cervical dilation when the fetal head is at +2 station or greater, regardless of position, when the requirements for outlet vacuum extraction are not met. Midpelvic vacuum extraction is the application of the vacuum extractor when the fetal head is engaged but the leading point of the skull is above +2 station, regardless of position.

Prerequisites

(a) Appropriate occipital, midline application of vacuum cup;
(b) Analgesia
  • Pudendal nerve block,
  • Saddle block,
  • (Uncommonly) epidural anesthesia,
  • (Rarely) general anesthesia;
(c) Operator certainty of fetal station and position. Pelvic examination to establish the station, position, and deflection of the fetal head,
(d) Empty maternal bladder (Credé, recent voiding);
(e) Full cervical dilatation;
(f) Ruptured membranes.

Application

The same procedure as for outlet vacuum extraction is followed, with careful attention to avoiding displacement of the fetal head during cup application and to applying traction in the pelvic curve (Figs. 4.7–4.11).

Discussion and Conclusions

The vacuum extractor is a particularly useful device for assisted vaginal delivery. It is, however, not without the potential for both fetal and maternal injury. European literature has favored the use of the vacuum extractor in many more clinical settings than has been popular in the United States. While the use of vacuum extraction for fetal distress and in cases of incomplete cervical dilatation is discussed at length in the literature, such applications have few, if any, American supporters. Clinical enthusiasm for the vacuum extractor has been variable in the last decade. The device is an important addition to the obstetrical armamentarium, but it must be treated with the respect due any surgical instrument.

Other than its ease in initial application, the vacuum extractor has an advantage over forceps in that rotation of the fetal head from anterior oblique and transverse positions is generally automatic, although at times it is assisted by finger pressure provided by the operator. The device is less successful in the conversion of occiput posterior presentations. In the delivery of the second, cephalic presentation twin, the vacuum extractor is often particularly helpful in prompt delivery via the flaccid, previously dilated birth canal. In addition, the vacuum extractor has an important clinical role in *trials* of instrumental delivery, especially when heavy cranial molding/caput succedaneum obscures clinical landmarks. In general, the vacuum extractor can be applied without major anesthesia and is less traumatic to the mother than forceps. However, fetal injuries are more common with vacuum extraction than with forceps applications although the majority of these are insignificant scalp ecchymoses and cephalhematomas (22).

Attention to detail is critical in avoidance of complications. In vacuum extractions, the cup needs to be positioned as closely as possible over the fetal occiput (Fig. 4.3) to assure adequate traction without extension of the fetal head. Also it is important to be certain that maternal tissues (cervical edge, lateral vaginal side wall) are not included within the grasp of the cup or else potentially serious maternal injuries will occur. Finally, care must be taken to avoid "popping" the cup from the fetal head or maintaining continuous traction/vacuum for an excessive period of time (i.e. >25 minutes) or else serious and potentially fatal fetal scalp injuries can be produced.

Comparison of Vacuum Extraction to Forceps

For American practitioners the principal question with the vacuum extractor is not whether the device works, but rather whether vacuum extraction has an acceptably low level of complications or any advantage(s) over alternative means of delivery, namely cesarean section or forceps. In general, forceps are more traumatic to the mother than vacuum extraction (17, 22). Vacuum extraction, however, is not necessarily benign (22, 51) (Tables 4.8 and 4.9). If the vacuum extractor is applied for too long a period of time or if not applied with careful attention to detail and technique of traction, serious fetal scalp injuries can result. Its very ease of use and apparent safety make vacuum extraction dangerous in poorly trained hands. On the other hand, vacuum extraction is easier to train personnel to use and the application of the cup is less critical in terms of exact anatomic positioning than with forceps blades.

Outlet Procedures

These are the simplest of assisted delivery procedures. Usually such interventions are necessary due to maternal exhaustion or inability to finally expel the infant when regional anesthesia has been administered. By definition, in such settings the fetal head has reached the pelvic floor and, usually, minimal assistance is necessary. Episiotomy may or may not be required, depending upon perineal anatomy as the fetal head crowns. Vacuum extraction has little to offer for outlet delivery. If a metal cup extraction is applied, a chignon will be raised with the attendant (albeit temporary) changes and a small risk of scalp injury exists. The Kobayashi extractor has been suggested for such applications. Our experience with the silastic device as an outlet instrument has been disappointing, as bending or distortion of the cup margin with loss of suction is common as the head crowns. In general, forceps are preferable for low or outlet assistance. True outlet forceps are atraumatic to the fetus and can virtually always be applied under pudendal block in a cooperative patient unless epidural anesthesia is already present. In sum, vacuum extraction has little advantage over forceps in outlet procedures, except it may be applied with less, and in some cases, no anesthesia.

Fetal Distress

While there is extensive European literature on the use of vacuum extraction in fetal distress, such applications are rare in the United States. Fetal distress with an undilated cervix is best managed by cesarean section. In unusual clinical settings with multiparous patients, the vacuum extractor can be applied at 7 cm or more when fetal distress is present but cephalopelvic disproportion is not an issue. With coordinated maternal expulsive efforts, delivery can occur more rapidly than cesarean section can be performed. However, if such a procedure is elected, concomitant preparations for cesarean delivery should be initiated. If the extraction is either lengthy or impossible, abdominal delivery is performed. In instances of fixed fetal bradycardias, forceps are almost always preferable to vacuum for most American practitioners due to experience and training of the accoucheur, the speed with which the instrument can be obtained, and the fact that no specialized additional apparatus, such as a suction pump, or assembly of disarticulated parts is necessary.

Trial of Instrumental Delivery

In this setting, the vacuum extractor has great potential application. The vacuum extractor is more easily applied than forceps in the midpelvis. There is clearly less maternal trauma with midpelvic vacuum extraction than midpelvic forceps delivery (23) (Table 4.8). Fetal damage of different types can occur with both instruments. Scalp injuries such as chignon or cephalhematoma are more frequent with the vacuum extractor while lacerations and ecchymoses are more common with forceps operations (Table 4.9). Also, neonatal jaundice occurs with greater frequency following vacuum extraction than with forceps (Table 4.3). Maternal injuries are more likely if forceps have been chosen. Serious fetal scalp injuries are rare with vacuum extraction *if* careful attention has been paid to the details of vacuum cup application and the technique of traction.

The vacuum extractor has a potential advantage in trials of vaginal delivery, as undiagnosed disproportion is the most dangerous

Table 4.8.   Maternal complications: 256 vacuum extractions with Malmström-type rigid metal cup versus 300 forceps deliveries[a]

	Vacuum Extraction	Forceps	P
Cervical lacerations	10 (3.9%)[b]	18 (6%)	NS[c]
Vaginal lacerations	27 (10.5%)[b]	71 (23.7%)	<0.001
Third-degree lacerations	41 (16%)	69 (23%)	<0.03
Fourth-degree lacerations	48 (18.7%)[b]	70 (23.3%)	NS

[a]Reprinted with permission from The American College of Obstetricians and Gynecologists (From Broekhuizen FF, Washington JM, Johnson F, Hamilton PR. Vacuum extraction versus forceps delivery: indications and complications, 1979 to 1984. Obstet Gynecol 1987; 69:338–342).
[b]Associated in six cases with failure of forceps.
[c]NS, not significant.

possibility in midpelvic arrest. Cephalopelvic disproportion as a cause of dystocia must never be overcome by *accouchement forcé*. The vacuum extractor has an inherent safety factor, as tractions exceeding 14–15 kg will in general break the suction. Much greater force is necessary to cause forceps blades to slip. In the hands of a highly experienced accoucheur, the forceps are probably equally as safe as the vacuum extractor. However, the built-in limitation of force with the extractor favors its use for many practitioners in trials of operative delivery. If station cannot be made *with the first traction effort* using the vacuum extractor, then forceps *should not* be applied, except in highly selected cases by experienced practitioners. The trial should be terminated and cesarean delivery performed.

Rotational Deliveries

This area is controversial. Certain rotational deliveries are best performed by forceps. This is especially true if the presentation is OP or obliquely posterior and anterior rotation is necessary to avoid unnecessary force during delivery. Vacuum extraction may occasionally

Table 4.9.   Perinatal complications: 256 vacuum extractions with Malmström-type rigid metal cup versus 300 forceps deliveries[a]

	Vacuum Extraction	Forceps	P
Cephalhematoma	10 (3.9%)	13 (4.3%)	NS[b]
Neonatal jaundice	73 (28.5%)	51 (17%)	<0.01
Skin ecchymoses/abrasions	113 (44.1%)	89 (29.5%)	<0.001
Subconjunctival hemorrhage	4 (1.5%)	13 (4.3%)	NS
Shoulder dystocia	8 (3.1%)	1 (0.3%)	<0.01
Mortality	1 (0.4%)	1 (0.3%)	NS
Seizures	1 (0.4%)	2 (0.6%)	NS

[a]Reprinted with permission from The American College of Obstetricians and Gynecologists (From Broekhuizen FF, Washington, JM, Johnson F, Hamilton, PR. Vacuum extraction versus forceps delivery: indications and complications, 1979 to 1984. Obstet Gynecol 1987; 69:338–342).
[b]NS, not significant.

suffice in posterior presentations, but the special "posterior" cup of Bird is usually required to achieve an acceptable application (2). With traction, "autorotation" does occur with vacuum extraction and can be assisted by finger pressure of the accoucheur (22).

REFERENCES

1. Simpson JR. On a suction tractor or new mechanical power as a substitute for forceps in tedious labours. Edinburgh Monthly J Med Sci 1849; 32:556–558.
2. Chalmers JA. The ventouse: the obstetric vacuum extractor. Chicago: Year Book, 1971.
3. Sjöstedt JE. The vacuum extractor and forceps in obstetrics: a clinical study. Acta Obstet Gynecol Scand 1967; 46(suppl 10):3–208.
4. Malmström T. The vacuum extractor. An obstetrical instrument and the parturiometer, a tokographic device. Acta Obstet Gynecol Scand 1957; 36(suppl 3):7–87.
5. Malmström T, Jansson I. Use of the vacuum extractor. Clin Obstet Gynecol 1965; 8:898–913.
6. Thiery M. Obstetric vacuum extraction. Obstet Gynecol Annu 1985; 14:73–111.
7. Goodall JR. The caput succedaneum: A hinderance to labour. J Obstet Gynaecol Br Emp 1933; 40:1021–1023.
8. Saling E, Hartung M. Analyses of tractive forces during the application of vacuum extraction. J Perinat Med 1973; 1:245–251.
9. Landgren L. The causes of foetal head moulding and labour. Acta Obstet Gynecol Scand 1960; 39:46–62.
10. Halme J, Ekbladh L. The vacuum extractor for obstetric delivery. Clin Obstet Gynaecol 1982; 25:167–175.
11. Mishell D, Kelly JV. The obstetrical forceps and the vacuum extractor: an assessment of their compressive force. Obstet Gynecol 1962; 19:204–206.
12. Rosa P. Defense de l'extraction par ventouse. Brux Med 1955; 35:1590–1597.
13. Moolgaoker AS, Ahmed SOS, Payne PR. A comparison of different methods of instrumental delivery based on electronic measurements of compression and traction. Obstet Gynecol 1979; 54:299–309.
14. Thiery M, VanKets H, Derom R. Recording of tractive power in vacuum extraction. J Perinat Med 1973; 1:291–292.
15. Roman I, Dinca G. Contributions to the augmentation of vacuum extraction in obstetrical practice. Rum Med Rev 1966; 20:74–81.
16. Malmström T. The vacuum extractor. Triangle 1962; 5:300–306.
17. Vacca W, Grant A, Wyatt G, Chalmers I. Portsmouth operative delivery trial: a comparison of vacuum extraction and forceps delivery. Br J Obstet Gynaecol 1983; 90:1107–1112.
18. Bird GC. The importance of flexion in vacuum extractor delivery. Br J Obstet Gynaecol 1976; 83:194–200.
19. Duchon MA, De Mund MA, Brown RH. Laboratory comparison of modern vacuum extractors. Obstet Gynecol 1988; 71:155–158.
20. Bird GC. The use of the vacuum extractor. Clin Obstet Gynaecol 1982; 9:641–661.
21. Apuzzio JJ, Pelosi MA, Ganesh VV. Fetal heart bradycardia associated with the vacuum extractor: a case report. J Reprod Med 1984; 29:496–497.
22. Broekhuizen FF, Washington JM, Johnson F, Hamilton PR. Vacuum extraction versus forceps delivery: indications and complications, 1979 to 1984. Obstet Gynecol 1987; 69:338–342.
23. Greis JB, Bieniarz J, Scommegna A. Comparison of maternal and fetal effects of vacuum extraction with forceps or cesarean deliveries. Obstet Gynecol 1981; 57:571–577.
24. Lasbrey AH, Orchard CD, Crichton D. A study of the relative merits and scope for vacuum extraction as opposed to forceps delivery. S Afr J Obstet Gynaecol 1964; 2:1–3.
25. Galvan BJ, Broekhuizen FF. Obstetric

vacuum extraction. J Obstet Gynecol Nurs 1987; 16:242–248.

26. Plauché WC. Fetal cranial injuries related to delivery with a Malmström vacuum extractor. Obstet Gynecol 1979; 53:750–757.

27. Plauché WC. Subgaleal hematoma: A complication of instrumental delivery. JAMA 1980; 244:1597–1598.

28. Rosemann GWE. Vacuum extraction of premature infants. S Afr J Obstet Gynaecol 1969; 7:10–12.

29. Witter FR. Soft-cup vacuum extractors safely assist normal deliveries. Contemp Obstet Gynecol 1985; 26(suppl):109–119.

30. Berkus MD, Ramamurthy RS, O'Conner PS, Brown K, Hayashi RH. Cohort study of silastic obstetric vacuum cup deliveries: I. Safety of the instrument. Obstet Gynecol 1985; 66:503–509.

31. Dell DL, Sightler SE, Plauché WC. Soft cup vacuum extraction: a comparison of outlet delivery. Obstet Gynecol 1985; 66:624–628.

32. Sennett ES, Fallis GB. Vacuum extraction: use in a small rural hospital. Can Med Assoc J 1983; 129:575–577.

33. Maryniak GM, Frank JB. Clinical assessment of the Kobayashi vacuum extractor. Obstet Gynecol 1984; 64:431–435.

34. Jackson U, Lanzara B, Rawlinson K, Chao S. Clinical experience with a soft silicone obstetric vacuum extractor [Abstract 357]. Society of Perinatal Obstetricians Seventh Annual Meeting, Lake Buena Vista, FL, February 5–7, 1987.

35. Hammarström M, Csemiczky G, Belfrage P. Comparison between the conventional Malmström extractor and a new extractor with silastic cup. Acta Obstet Gynecol Scand 1986; 65:791–792.

36. Bird GC. Modification of Malmström's vacuum extractor. Br Med J 1969; 3:526.

37. Wood JF. An evaluation of a new plastic disposable vacuum extractor cup. J Am Osteopath Assoc 1969; 66:1251–54.

38. Paul RH, Staisch KJ, Pine SN. The "new" vacuum extractor. Obstet Gynecol 1973; 41:800-802.

39. O'Grady JP. Clinical management of twins. Contemp Obstet Gynecol 1987; 29:126–145.

40. Solomons E. Delivery of the head with the Malmström vacuum extractor during cesarean section. Obstet Gynecol 1962; 19:201–203.

41. Bercovici B. Use of the vacuum extractor for head delivery at cesarean section. Isr J Med Sci 1980; 16:201–203.

42. Pelosi MA, Apuzzio, J. Use of the soft, silicone obstetric vacuum cup for the delivery of the fetal head at cesarean section. J Reprod Med 1984; 29:289–292.

43. Boehm FH. Vacuum extraction during cesarean section. South Med J 1985; 78:1502.

44. Chamberlain G. Forceps and vacuum extraction. Clin Obstet Gynaecol 1980; 7:511–527.

45. Altaras M, Potashnik G, Ben-Adereth N, Leventhal H. The use of vacuum extraction in cases of cord prolapse during labor. Am J Obstet Gynecol 1974; 118:824–830.

46. Fahmy K, Ghali A. The place of vacuum extraction in prolapsed pulsating cord. Aust NZ J Obstet Gynaecol 1977; 17:36–39.

47. Brat T. Indications for and results of the use of the "ventouse obstetricale" (a ten year study). J Obstet Gynaecol Br Commonw 1965; 72:883–888.

48. Inman SE. The use of the vacuum extractor in the first stage of labour. J Obstet Gynaecol Br Commonw 1969; 76:354–358.

49. Roberts IF, Stone M. Fetal hemorrhage: Complication of vacuum extractor after fetal blood sampling. Am J Obstet Gynecol 1978; 132:109.

50. Thiery M. Fetal hemorrhage following blood samplings and use of vacuum extractor [Letter to the editor]. Am J Obstet Gynecol 1979; 134:231.

51. Bliennow G, Svenningsen NW, Gustafson B, Sunden B, Cronquist S. Neonatal and prospective follow-up study of infants delivery by vacuum extraction (VE). Acta Obstet Gynecol Scand 1977; 56:189–194.

5

Complications and Birth Injuries

Obstetrics is not one of the exact sciences, and in our penury of truth we ought to be accurate in our statements, generous in our doubts, tolerant in our convictions. . . .

JAMES YOUNG SIMPSON, 1875 (1)

Forceps Operations

Maternal Birth Injuries

Maternal injuries are commonly associated with the process of instrumental delivery. As Table 5.1 indicates, the reported incidence of complications is extremely variable. Most maternal complications consist of birth canal lacerations, episiotomy extensions, and associated hemorrhage. The majority of these complications are of minor clinical consequence although some are severe or serious. The more significant injuries are avoidable by simple caution, for example, declining to perform heroic procedures or use excessive force. In considering such injuries, it is best to divide them into the categories of acute events and complications (Table 5.2).

As the mother requires assistance during delivery, either she is incapable of expelling the fetus or overwhelming reasons such as fetal or maternal distress necessitate prompt delivery. In either circumstance, the lower vaginal tissues have not been subjected to the ironing out and slow progressive distention that normally occurs as the pre-

Table 5.1. Complications of Forceps Delivery, Selected Series

	Dunlop (2) N = 292	Taylor (3) N = 31	Cooke (4) N = 427	Danforth & Ellis (5) N = 1000	Cosgrove & Weaver (6) N = 1000	Gilstrap et al. (7) N = 234
Postpartum hemorrhage	3	26	6.7	4.4		
Cervical lacerations	1.4	22.6	9.8	19.6	2.9	
Episiotomy complications	1				16.2	
Foot drop					0.1	
Endometritis	0.7					
Ruptured uterus					0.1	
UTI[a]	0.3					
Bladder injury					0.3	
Urinary retention		16	4.2			
Coccyx fracture	0.3		0.47		0.1	
Hematoma pelvis	0.3					
Vaginal lacerations		13	6.7		4.0	62
3rd degree tear		3.2			3.5	
Rectovaginal fistula		3.2				
Puerperal fever		13				
Sphincter laceration			10			
Complete tear			6.7		2.5	
Sulcus tears			21			
Multiple vaginal tears			0.4			
% of mothers with one or more complications		51.6	19			

[a]UTI, urinary tract infection.

senting part descends. Thus, there is some degree of soft tissue dystocia to be overcome whenever instrumental delivery is performed. Further, extraction from higher station requires an angle of pull that heavily pressures the perineal body and posterior vaginal vault. These pressures will often produce a midline perineal laceration if an episiotomy is not made first. However, in multiparous women or in the occasional nullipara with marked vaginal relaxation, or in whom the perineum can be ironed out, episiotomy may not be required if extraction is both slow and gentle. It is unclear whether episiotomy predisposes to rectal laceration. The extension of the episiotomy into the rectal spincter (third degree) or further posterior into the rectum itself (fourth degree) is not uncommon. Such extensions are no longer necessarily considered an obstetrical disaster or indicative of an inexcusably poor technique. However, these injuries increase maternal morbidity,

Table 5.2.   Possible Maternal Injuries from Forceps Delivery

Acute injuries
   Birth canal lacerations (vagina, cervix)
   Episiotomy extensions (rectal injury)
   Bladder, paraurethral, or urethral injuries
   Vaginal hematoma
   Uterine rupture
   Rupture of the symphysis pubis
   Fracture or subluxation of coccyx
   Nerve injuries
      Sural
      Iliac
   Vessel injuries
Chronic and/or related complications
   Infection
      Cellulitis or local abscess
      Necrotizing fascitis
   Uterine atony
   Anemia, hemorrhagic shock, vascular collapse
   Fistula formation
      Rectovaginal
      Vesicovaginal
      Vesicouterine
   Bladder atony, inability to void
   Perineal scarring, dyspareunia
   Thrombosis, embolism

carry a risk of secondary infection, and can break down with fistula formation for an overall risk approaching 1%. It is claimed that the mediolateral episiotomy avoids such rectal injuries. However, this incision creates other problems of its own. Mediolateral episiotomies are extremely painful to the patient. Further, with healing, distortion of the perineum and accompanying dyspareunia is not uncommon. It should be noted, however, that the data on these points are largely anecdotal and good studies are rare. Clinically most patients are more comfortable if midline rather than mediolateral episiotomy has been performed. Even with fourth degree lacerations rectovaginal fistulae are uncommon if there is prompt identification of the injury and anatomic repair of the rectal defect.

The operator should not labor to avoid episiotomy when instrumental delivery is performed. A surgical incision of the perineum is more easily repaired and likely will heal with less scarring than a jagged laceration. However, the perineum should be incised only when necessary and while it is under tension, both to minimize blood loss and to better judge the extent of the incision that is required.

The importance of avoiding periurethral and anterior vaginal vault lacerations is not adequately emphasized. Failure to apply traction in Carus' curve, rapid accouchement over a firm or unyielding perineum, or uncontrolled descent of the fetal head results in peri-urethral lacerations. Such injuries appear as linear cracks in the thin tissue lying to either side of the clitoris or urethra. These injuries are difficult to repair and can bleed profusely. Following repair, many women will be unable to void and either intermittent or chronic catheterization is required. On occasion such lacerations heal with scarring, resulting in chronic dyspareunia.

The most serious vaginal vault lacerations are those that involve the pudendal artery, leading to the formation of a hematoma. The pudendal artery can be lacerated or avulsed during spontaneous uninstrumented delivery with or without a history of pudendal nerve block. Such hematomas can be serious and commonly require surgical exploration, vaginal packing, and/or blood transfusion. Uncommonly, if neglected, rapidly developing hematomas lead to vascular collapse and hemorrhagic shock. The presenting symptom is unremitting vaginal pain accompanied by a progressive gross unilateral swelling of the labia.

Infection is surprisingly uncommon in obstetric injuries considering the frequency of open wounds, surgical incisions of the perineum, spontaneous lacerations that occur during pregnancy, and their obvious contamination by the ubiquitous genital tract bacterial flora. Presumably it is the extensive blood supply of the birth canal that makes infection uncommon. Infection, if it does occur, is usually minor. Infrequently an episiotomy site or laceration repair will break down due to infection. Infection rarely can be life-threatening if either puerperal septicemia, septic pyelonephritis, necrotizing fasciitis, or clostridial myonecrosis develop (8, 9). Fortunately, all of these serious complications are rare. Necrotizing fasciitis is the most feared, albeit rare, of these complications. This disorder is a progressive necrosis of tissue tracking along fascial planes (9–13). The causative organism is the Group A, B-hemolytic streptococcus alone or in combination with anaerobic bacteria (*Bacteroides* species) or, less commonly, Streptococcus with bacteria other than anaerobes or *Enterobacteriaceae* (11). The patient commonly has experienced extensive perineal lacerations with repair (9). The presenting symptom is a complaint of severe vaginal pain and there is a characteristic "dishwater-colored" wound discharge. Diagnosis by inspection alone is unreliable. Examination of the repair site notes variable skin changes (9). Localized tenderness may occur but, as the disease progresses, the area often becomes progressively anesthetic (12). Surgical exploration of the perineum is indicated in the presence of skin erythema or edema beyond the immediate episiotomy site/perineal laceration, if severe systemic signs are present or if apparent infection does not promptly respond to antibiotic therapy (9). Separation of skin from deep fascia and failure of the fascia to bleed when incised strongly suggest the correct diagnosis. Treatment is rapid and aggressive debridement of all devitalized tissue. General supportive measures and systemic, wide-spectrum antibiotics are also indicated. However, prompt surgical removal of all devitalized tissue is the first priority. Successful surgical treatment may require extensive dissection into the perineum. The surgeon must be aggressive, as this condition is life-threatening.

Infection reaching the deep fascia can produce myonecrosis, commonly by clostridial infection (9). Myonecrosis can also result from neglected necrotizing fasciitis, accompanying invasion of deep fascia. The predisposing factors are tissue destruction and wound contamination with bowel flora. The most common organism is the Gram-positive obligate anaerobic bacteria, *Clostrididium perfringens* (*welchii*) (8). Severe pain, systemic signs (tachycardia, hypotension, restlessness), rapid progression, and wound crepitation are classic signs of clostridial infection (8). A smear of the wound reveals Gram-positive rods. Treatment is similar to that for necrotizing fasciitis with aggressive surgical debridement and antibiotic therapy. High dose penicillin and wide, even radical, incision of all involved tissue is required. Polyvalent antitoxin and hyperbaric oxygen are secondary measures, the former of uncertain benefit.

Rarely, uterine rupture occurs with a forceps operation. The most common cause is uterine perforation during attempted insertion of a forceps blade. Loss of station, vaginal bleeding, maternal shock, or fetal distress are the usual signs if rupture has occurred. Prompt surgical exploration and repair are indicated.

Infant Birth Injuries

The outcome of delivery, whether spontaneous or instrumental, is not invariably normal. Minor abrasions, ecchymoses, and cephalhematomas are common in the delivery process and are of no long-term clinical significance. It is the responsibility of the accoucheur to be certain that the risk to mother and infant in any delivery, operative or spontaneous, is minimized by the most meticulous attention to indications and technique. Serious birth injury is uncommon but can result in permanent neonatal damage. In 1984, birth injuries caused 8.9 deaths per 100,000 livebirths, falling to eighth among leading causes of neonatal loss (14). Morbidity is even a larger issue that tends to be obscured when mortality statistics are presented. For every neonatal death assigned to birth trauma as many as 20 surviving neonates experience a major birth injury (15, 16). Birth injury has both major economic and social costs and, of course, medicolegal risk. However, neither spontaneous vaginal delivery nor cesarean section will guarantee an infant that is free from traumatic injury, and it is not possible to perform instrumental delivery without some maternal and fetal risk of injury. In assessing the risk or benefit from any obstetric intervention, both maternal and fetal costs must be weighed.

Our terminology in this regard is unfortunate. Under the term "birth injury" we generally include all significant neonatal abnormalities identified following birth. Some of these are due to direct trauma but the majority result from developmental anomalies of the fetus and/ or prematurity (17). For the purposes of this discussion, *birth injury* is best defined as injury occurring during the process of parturition resulting from the mechanical forces of instrumental delivery, producing hemorrhage, tissue injury, or alteration of organ function (16).

The factors associated with birth-related injuries are multiple (Table 5.3) and involve difficulties in fetal extraction, problems of dystotic labor, and fetal congenital anomalies. Instrumental delivery is frequently associated with one or more of these factors as a fellow traveler. The task for the reviewer is to separate, if possible, associated events from truly etiologic ones.

Mortality and morbidity at birth are largely dependent upon gestational age (18, 19). In preterm infants, respiratory distress, perinatal asphyxia/hypoxia, intracranial hemorrhage, and infection are

Table 5.3.   Factors Predisposing to Birth-Associated Injuries

Fetal macrosomia
Premature delivery
Abnormal Labor
  Precipitous labor
  Dystocia/prolonged labor
Obstetric procedures
  Internal version and extraction
  Forceps or vacuum extraction
  Scalp sampling/scalp electrodes
  Umbilical vessel blood sampling
  Amniocentesis
Malpresentation
  Face/brow
  Breech
  Occiput posterior
Fetal anomalies
  Hydrops fetalis
  Hydrocephalus
  Sacrococcygeal teratomas
  Cystic hygromas
  Goiter
Multiple gestations

common events. In contrast, in term infants respiratory difficulties are uncommon and congenital abnormalities of various types represent an increased percentage of the infants found to be damaged. It is also true that term infants, particularly macrosomic term infants, are more likely to experience mechanical or iatrogenic birth trauma by instrumental or assisted delivery (20).

The relationship between birth asphyxia and trauma is complex. The already asphyxiated neonate may be at greater risk of injury either because of changes in muscle tone or existing hypoxic/ischemic injury or because of the haste of the accoucheur in achieving delivery if distress occurs with the stress of labor (21). In growth-retarded neonates, either the small size of the infant or malpresentation (e.g., breech) predispose to a more difficult or traumatic delivery. Also trauma itself causes shock with resultant anoxic/ischemic damage to tissues. Some injuries are occult and often left to the scrutiny of the pathologist in the limited number of neonates coming to necropsy (21, 22). For example, a primary diagnosis of intracranial birth trauma may not be made during life even with the assistance of modern methods of evaluation. The true lesion may be identified only at necropsy.

The most frequent birth-associated injuries are clavicular fractures and palsies of the facial nerve and brachial plexus (Table 5.4). By no means are all of these associated with instrumental delivery, as some occur in spontaneous vaginal deliveries and can even be found in infants delivered by cesarean section. Other lesions are associated with forceps delivery (Table 5.5) or vacuum extraction (Tables 4.8 and 4.9). The major categories of injury for both forceps and vacuum extractor operations are individually reviewed in the following section.

Cephalhematoma

Diagnosis. A cephalhematoma consists of a collection of blood under the scalp in a newborn infant (Fig. 5.1). Cephalhematomas develop when the soft tissues of the scalp are buffeted back and forth

Table 5.4. Incidence of Birth Trauma, Selected Series[a]

Author	Clavicular Fracture	Facial Nerve Injury	Brachial Plexus Injury
		Injury	
Madsen (23)	7.0/1000 (N = 726)		
Rubin (24)	2.7/1000 (N = 43)	1.3/1000 (N = 21)	1.2/1000 (N = 18)
Tan (25)			0.63/1000 (N = 57)
Gordon et al. (26)			1.89/1000 (N = 59)
Cohen & Otto (27)	7.1/1000 (N = 24)		
Levine et al. (20)	2.0/1000 (N = 28)	7.5/1000 (N = 104)	2.6/1000 (N = 36)

[a]Modified from Levine MG, Holroyde J, Woods JR, Siddiqui TA, MacHenry S, Miodovnik M. Birth trauma: incidence and predisposing factors. Obstet Gynecol 1984; 63:792–795.

Table 5.5. Neonatal Complications of Forceps Application

Cephalhematoma
Subgaleal hematoma
Shoulder girdle dystocia and brachial plexus injury
Retinal hemorrhage
Ecchymoses, lacerations, and subcutaneous fat necrosis
Intracranial hemorrhage/injury
Skull and facial fractures
Spinal cord injury
Fractures (clavicle, humerus, femur)
Facial nerve palsy
Rare complications
Mortality

over the more rigid underlying bone during spontaneous or instrumentally assisted delivery (14). The lesion then results from an effusion of fetal blood beneath the pericranium due to laceration of the bridging subperiosteal vessels. On palpation cephalhematomas are usually fluctuant and often bordered by an elevated ridge, giving a false sensation of a central bony depression (14).

Cephalhematomas are to be separated from caput succedaneum and subaponeurotic hemorrhages. In caput succedaneum, the effusion is entirely *independent* of the periosteum of the bone and consists of serum. There is no overlying discoloration. Caput succedaneum is present at birth, which is not invariably true for cephalhematoma. Also, caput succedaneum resolves more rapidly than hematoma. In cephalhematomas, the swelling is contained by the suture line, which usually sharply delimits the lesion. The bleeding usually occurs over one or both parietal bones. Lesions over the occiput are less common and over the frontal bones, rare. Clinically, large cephalhematomas may be difficult to distinguish from caput succedaneum.

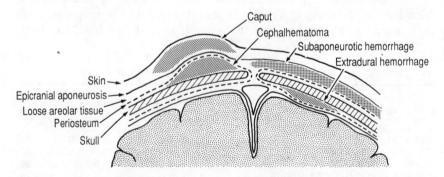

Figure 5.1.   Sites of cranial and extradural hemorrhage in the newborn cranium. (From Pape WE, Wigglesworth, JS. Haemorrhage, Ischaemia and the Perinatal Brain. Philadelphia: JB Lippincott, 1979.

Table 5.6. Incidence of Cephalhematoma

Author	Instrumentation/Comments	Incidence (%)
Instrumental delivery		
Munsat et al. (28)	All	2.7
Churchill et al. (29)	Midpelvic rotation, no rotation	32.7
Cooke (4)	Midpelvic rotation, no rotation	5.4
Schenker & Serr (30)	All	5.0
Widen et al. (31)	All	0
Healy et al. (32)	Kielland forceps	7
Vacca et al. (33)	All	5.2
Benkus et al. (34)	All	4.7
Spontaneous		
Churchill et al. (29)		2.44
Yasunaga & Rivera (35)		0.32

Subgaleal hematomas are much more serious lesions where the hemorrhage is not confined to a limited potential space and is accompanied often by clinical signs and symptoms of vascular collapse, variable scalp fluctuance, and discoloration (see discussion of cephalhemata under "Complications of Vacuum Extraction"). Such subperiosteal bleeding may be slow and the swelling may not develop until hours or even days postpartum.

Incidence. Cephalhematomas occur in approximately 5% of instrumental deliveries. The lesion is significantly more frequent with midforceps and vacuum extraction than in spontaneous delivery (Table 5.6). Also associated with an increased likelihood of scalp injury are nulliparity and prolonged labor (Table 5.7). Vacuum extraction is an additional important etiologic factor.

Comments. Cephalhematomas can be large and misdiagnosed as scalp edema (caput succedaneum). Occasionally, neonatal anemia or hyperbilirubinemia results from the hemorrhage and its subsequent resorption.

In the study of Churchill et al. (29) the fetal brain was apparently unaffected by the trauma that resulted in the cephalhematoma, as indicated by α-like electroencephalogram (EEG) rhythms at birth and a normal incidence of diffuse central nervous system disorders. Finally,

Table 5.7. Characteristics of Infants with Cephalhematoma[a]

90% were occiput anterior presentation
70% from primiparous pregnancy
63% forceps delivery (62% low; 2% mid)
47% prolonged labor (2nd stage)
  7% skull fracture
  4% low birth weight (<2500 g)
  4% premature (<36 weeks)

[a]Modified from Yasunaga S, Rivera R. Cephalhematoma in the newborn. Observations based on a review of 139 infants. Clin Pediatr 1974; 13:256–260.

there were no apparent attributable long-term neurologic sequelae. The treatment of cephalhematoma is conservative unless bleeding appears to be progressive. Hematomas should neither be needled nor surgically drained, as complete spontaneous reabsorption is the rule and instrumentation may introduce infection. Rarely, blood loss can be severe enough to require transfusion. Associated hyperbilirubinemia can require phototherapy. The cephalhematoma normally will resorb completely within 4 weeks. While aspiration is not advisable due to the risk of infection, both meningitis and septicemia have been reported with spontaneous infection without instrumentation. Calcification commonly occurs within the lesion but normally disappears within 3–6 months. Uncommonly, cystic defects may persist at the site of the hematoma for months or even years. Rarely, a scalp mass persists even into adulthood (14)—the cephalhematoma deformans of Schüller. There is an association between cephalhematomas and underlying skull fracture. In some series as many as 25–50% of cephalhematomas are accompanied by an underlying fracture (36). However, in the experience of most clinicians this estimate is much too high. This contention is strengthened by data from the study of Zelson (37), who reported a much lower incidence (5.4%) of associated fractures—a number much more in accord with clinical experience. If a fracture with a wide diastasis is present, exploration to prevent the eventual development of a leptomeningeal cyst may be required as an underlying dural laceration with leakage of cerebral spinal fluid can be present.

Subgaleal (Subaponeurotic) Hematoma

Diagnosis.   A subgaleal hematoma is a collection of blood in the loose connective tissue in the potential space between the periosteum of the cranial bones (paracranium) and the galea aponeurotica (epicranial aponeurosis) (38) (Fig. 5.1). The diagnosis is suspected in instances of difficult delivery if unusual fluctuation or discoloration of the scalp is observed. The presentation may be neonatal vascular collapse or shock at an indeterminate period following delivery.

Incidence.   The incidence is estimated to be 4/10,000 deliveries. In a study of 123 cases, approximately 30% occurred spontaneously and less than 10% at cesarean section (38). The remainder were divided between cases of vacuum extraction or forceps delivery (Table 5.8).

Comments.   Subaponeurotic hematomas are rare injuries but represent a potentially life-threatening condition that requires prompt identification and vigorous treatment.

Table 5.8.   Subgaleal Hematoma: Mode of Delivery in 123 Cases[a]

	No.	%
Spontaneous	35	28.4
Forceps	17	13.8
Vacuum extraction	60	48.8
Cesarean section	11	8.9
Total	123	100.0

[a]From Plauché WC. Subgaleal hematoma: a complication of instrumental delivery. JAMA 1980; 244:1597–1598. Copyright 1980, American Medical Association.

Shoulder Girdle Dystocia and Brachial Plexus Injury

Diagnosis.   Shoulder girdle dystocia is a condition of disproportion that occurs when the fetal bisachromial diameter attempts to enter the maternal pelvis but cannot negotiate the pelvic brim (the obstetric conjugate) (39–46). Obstruction occurs due to the relative dimensions between the fetal thorax and the maternal pelvis. The anterior shoulder cannot pass beneath the pubic symphysis although delivery of the head occurs and the fetal arms are normally positioned. A common clinical observation is *cranial recoil*, a characteristic rapid retrograde movement of the fetal head following spontaneous or assisted delivery ("turtle sign"). Subsequent bimanual traction on the head is unavailing or difficult. Successful extraction avoiding fetal or maternal injury requires knowledge of pelvic anatomy, dispatch, and *sang-froid*.

Incidence.   The occurrence of shoulder dystocia is closely tied to fetal size (29, 41, 44–47). In general, the incidence of dystocia rises rapidly when the fetus exceeds 4000 g (Tables 5.9 and 5.10). The overall incidence is approximately 5/1000 deliveries (Table 5.11). It must be emphasized that shoulder dystocia is certainly underreported. Only cases requiring special manipulations or resulting in neonatal injury are reliably recorded. Many lesser instances occur which are not reflected in collected series. Problems with shoulder delivery are much more likely to occur when instrumental delivery is combined with slow progress in the second stage of labor (Table 5.11). The over-

Table 5.9.   Risk Factors for Shoulder Dystocia

Fetal macrosomia (>4000 g)
Prolonged second stage and/or slow descent of the fetal head
Midforceps/midpelvic vacuum extraction
Gestational or insulin-requiring diabetes
Postmature pregnancy
Multiparity
Maternal obesity
Prior macrosomic infant or prior shoulder dystocia delivery

Table 5.10. Shoulder Dystocia Incidence: Type of Delivery and Fetal Weight[a]

Type of Delivery	<Fetal Weight (g)>	Incidence Shoulder Dystocia	%
Vertex/vaginal	<4000	6/7836	0.07
PSS + MPD[b]	<4000	6/360	1.6
Vertex/vaginal	≥4000	8/638	1.2
PSS + MPD	≥4000	13/56	23.0

[a]Reprinted with permission from The American College of Obstetricians and Gynecologists From Benedetti TJ, Gabbe SG. Shoulder dystocia. A complication of fetal macrosomia and prolonged second stage of labor with midpelvic delivery. Obstet Gynecol 1978; 52:526–529.
[b]PSS, prolonged second stage of labor; MPD, midpelvic delivery.

all incidence of shoulder dystocia with unselected midforceps procedures is approximately 4% (Table 5.12). However, if slow second stage progress, midpelvic delivery, and fetal macrosomia are present, the likelihood of shoulder dystocia approaches one in four (Table 5.10).

Comments. Shoulder dystocia is a potentially serious complication of delivery and prompt intervention is necessary. While an impacted shoulder is a potential risk in any vaginal delivery, it clearly occurs more frequently when fetal macrosomia, instrumental delivery, and slow second stage progress are combined. A number of procedures are described to reduce shoulder dystocia based on reducing the size of the fetal thorax, repositioning the fetal shoulders to a larger pelvic diameter, or changing pelvic diameter, or changing pelvic diameters by maternal reposition or even symphysiotomy (Table 5.13). In unusually severe cases, complete replacement of the fetal head with subsequent cesarean section has also been advocated (Zavanelli maneuver).

Shoulder dystocia is now uncommonly associated with fetal loss, but morbidity is a serious issue. In the combined series of Swartz (48), McCall (49), Seigworth (46), and Benedetti (42), in 220 cases of shoulder dystocia, 29 brachial plexus injuries (13.2%) were reported along with 14 fractures of the clavicle or humerus (6.4%) (see "Brachial Plexus Injury").

Avoidance of the complication is clearly desirable despite Shute's pronouncement that "... with shoulder dystocia there is neither prophecy nor prevention" (56). Avoidance of midpelvic vac-

Table 5.11. Occurrence of Shoulder Dystocia

Author	No. of Cases/Deliveries	<Incidence (%)>	(Deaths)/PNM[a]
Swartz (48)	31/20,599	0.15	(5) 161/1000
McCall (49)	105/16,000	0.63	(2) 198/1000
Seigworth (46)	51/13,491	0.38	(5) 98/1000
Benedetti and Gabbe (41)	33/9,864	0.37	(0)
Benedetti (42)	21/16,694	0.13	(0)

[a]PNM, perinatal mortality attributed to dystocia.

Table 5.12. Shoulder Dystocia Incidence: Association with Unselected Midpelvic Forceps Deliveries

Author	%
Hughey et al. (50)	3.9
Healy et al. (32)	4

uum extraction or forceps delivery in the setting of known fetal macrosomia and poor progress is prudent (42, 47). Ultrasonic evaluation of the fetus is helpful both for an estimation of weight and the determination of various ratios between head and body (57, 58, 59). If the transthoracic diameter at the level of the diaphragm exceeds the biparietal measurement by 1.4 cm, or the abdominal diameter exceeds the biparietal diameter by 1.5 cm, a greater likelihood for dystocia exists (59). However, these recommendations have not been sufficiently validated to serve as the sole basis for clinical management. Dependent upon clinical circumstances the practitioner can use these data to perform cesarean delivery, to conduct labor with avoidance of instrumental assistance planning prompt cesarean delivery if failure of descent occurs, or to conduct a vaginal trial, with preparations to treat shoulder dystocia if it occurs. A comparative study of clinical utility of any of these approaches has never been, and likely will never be, performed.

Brachial Plexus Injury (Erb's Palsy, Klumpke's Paralysis)

Diagnosis. The diagnosis of brachial plexus injury is by direct observation. The neonate fails to move one hand or arm in a normal fashion. The fifth and sixth cervical roots are most vulnerable. Damage to these nerves produces Duchenne/Erb's palsy, the "waiter's tip" deformity. The affected arm is rotated inward with extension and

Table 5.13. Procedures for Delivery in Shoulder Dystocia

Increase pelvic capacity: symphysiotomy (51)
Decrease fetal bisacromial size: clavicular fracture/cleidotomy (44)
Intrauterine replacement of fetal head (Zavanelli maneuver) (52)
Pressure to deliver anterior shoulder, anteriorly
    Fundal pressure (Kristeller technique) (39)
    Vectis expression, manual (Heery maneuver) or instrumental
    Suprapubic pressure (53)
    Posterior head pressure (Hibbard maneuver) (54)
    Maternal repositioning (MacRoberts maneuver and knee chest positioning) (55)
Fetal rotational maneuvers
    Corkscrew extraction (Woods maneuver and modifications) (40,43,46,48)
    Extraction of the posterior arm (45)
Instrumental delivery
    Vectis blade shoulder displacement
    Thoracic forceps application and rotation (Shute's maneuver) (56)

adduction. If the seventh and eighth and first thoracic roots are damaged, the forearm and hand are affected. If only the lower roots are damaged, only the hand is affected and the lesion is known as Klumpke's paralysis. The fifth cervical nerve root also gives rise to the phrenic nerve. Thus, respiratory difficulties may be observed in some neonates with concomitant brachial plexus injuries. An ipsilateral Horner's syndrome can be present with ptosis, miosis, and enophthalmos due to involvement of cervical sympathetic fibers of the first thoracic root. Weigert's palsy involves an Erb/Duchenne brachial plexus lesion combined with diaphragmatic paralysis (60). Rarely, spinal cord injuries can accompany brachial nerve palsies, presumably due to excessive nerve root traction. "Pseudo-Erb's" palsy is also possible due to injuries of the shoulder joint with tearing of the capsule, or fractures of the clavicle and fracture, dislocation, or detachment of the upper epiphysis of the humerus (14). In these circumstances, the neonate fails to move the involved extremity normally, giving rise to the erroneous suspicion of nerve injury.

Incidence. When all deliveries are included, the overall reported incidence is approximately 0.96/1000 live births (Table 5.14). Most cases occur in association with shoulder girdle dystocia or vaginal breech delivery. The injured infant is usually macrosomic, flaccid, and partially asphyxiated and thus more vulnerable to injury (14). In breech deliveries, the incidence of palsy is 175-fold greater than in cephalic presentations. Brachial plexus injury occurs in association with assisted delivery but is not directly due to cranial compression or repositioning but to problems of fetopelvic outlet disproportion (Table 5.15). The overall incidence with forceps deliveries is less than 1%.

Comments. Injuries to the brachial plexus are caused by trauma to the brachial nerve roots (60, 61, 62). The brachial plexus is a complex of nerves including the fifth, sixth, seventh, and eighth cervical and first and second thoracic nerve roots. The plexus is damaged principally by stretching, resulting in hemorrhage or edema into the nerve sheaths, compressing the fibers. In some instances there may be

Table 5.14. Incidence of Brachial Plexus Injury in Large Clinical Series

Author	N/total deliveries[a]	Incidence/1000 livebirths
Vassalos et al. (61)	169/66,149	2.50
Tan (25)	57/90,436	0.63
Gordon et al. (26)	59/31,700	1.89
Specht (62)	11/19,314	0.57
McFarland et al. (47)	106/210,947	0.50
Total	402/418,546	0.96

[a]Nonselected.

Table 5.15. Incidence of Brachial Plexus Injury with Forceps Delivery

Author	Injury	Type of Forceps Delivery	%
Cooke (4)	Erb's	Mid, with rotation	0.47
Schenker & Serr (30)	Erb's	Unspecified	0.4
Hughey et al. (50)	All	Mid, with rotation	1.5

rupture of the perineural sheath, accompanied by bleeding into the nerve trunk, associated with separation of the nerve fibers. In unusual cases complete avulsion of nerve roots occurs with injury to spinal gray matter. The plexus is usually damaged by lateral traction on the head in cases of shoulder dystocia or in breech presentation by downward traction on the shoulders and delivery for the aftercoming head. Complete recovery is the rule with 80% of injuries spontaneously regressing within 3–6 months. Klumpke's paralysis is uncommon, occurring in 2–3% of all injuries, and has a much poorer prognosis with only 40% showing complete recovery in 1 year. In the reviews of Levine et al. (20) and McFarland et al. (47) fetal macrosomia and poor progress in the second stage were important associations. As previously described, shoulder girdle dystocia, breech delivery, and maternal nulliparity are contributing factors.

Treatment in the newborn period is symptomatic with the aim of maintaining full range of motion to prevent contracture while awaiting recovery. Erb's palsy is usually managed with frequent range of motion exercises and diurnal splinting. Routine surgical exploration and attempts at repair are not indicated. Exploration may be indicated in selected neonates who fail to improve neurologically after 3–6 months of conservative therapy.

Ecchymoses, Lacerations, and Subcutaneous Fat Necrosis

Diagnosis. Neonatal soft tissue injuries are noted by direct clinical observation following birth. Ecchymoses or lacerations from forceps injuries occur on the fetal scalp or face, reflecting the sites of blade application. Areas of subcutaneous fat necrosis are irregular, firm, nonpitting lesions. The overlying skin may be colorless, red, or purple. No tenderness or erythema is present (63).

Incidence. Some bruising occurs in all spontaneous deliveries. Noninstrument-related fetal lacerations are at best rare. Rotational deliveries are more likely to result in lacerations than simple direct tractions unless unusual difficulty in blade insertion was present (Table 5.16).

Comments. Other than being cosmetically unpleasant, such injuries are of little consequence with the exception of occasional problems with neonatal jaundice from the reabsorption of hemoglobin

Table 5.16. Incidence of Neonatal Lacerations and Bruising Associated with Forceps Delivery

Author	Type of Delivery	<Lacerations (%)>	<Bruising (%)>
Munsat et al. (28)	All, unspecified	2.7	
Schenker & Serr (30)	All, unspecified	4.0	
Cooke (4)	Mid, no rotation	1.2	0.47
Healy et al. (32)	Rotation, non-Kielland	2.0	
	Kielland	3.0	

with extensive injury. Ecchymotic lesions are more likely to be forceps-related while lacerations are most commonly associated with either cesarean section (inadvertent scalpel injury) or rigid-cup vacuum extraction (scalp injury). In the latter instances, such injuries are avoidable by careful technique. Rarely, a laceration may require suturing or application of adhesive strips. Bruising or superficial ecchymoses resorb spontaneously within several days. The site should be kept clean and observed daily. Areas involving laceration or severe ecchymoses should be carefully examined to exclude underlying, occult fractures, hematomas, or other injuries. Areas of fat necrosis slowly soften and eventually resolve, although months may be required for complete resolution. Significant sequelae are rare.

Retinal Hemorrhage

Diagnosis. Retinal hemorrhages are diagnosed by direct ophthalmoscopic examination of the newborn. The neonate's eyes are dilated by mydriatic drops and the ocular fundus visualized by a trained examiner. Mechanical retraction of the eyelids by an assistant may be required for adequate evaluation.

Incidence. The literature reports a wide range of incidence for retinal hemorrhage for spontaneous and instrumentally assisted delivery (Table 5.17) (64–74). In a selected series of 4724 cases, the mean incidence of retinal hemorrhage in spontaneous deliveries was 27%. The rate of retinal hemorrhage occurring in forceps-delivered infants is not significantly different (29%). Cesarean section appears to be protective, with all authors reporting a low incidence (approximately 2%) when abdominal delivery is performed. There is general agreement that use of the vacuum extractor increases the rate of hemorrhage. Approximately 40% of infants delivered by vacuum extraction have retinal hemorrhage when careful direct ophthalmoscopy is performed.

Comment. Retinal hemorrhages are the most common ophthalmologic birth injury and are largely dependent upon the mode of assisted delivery. The majority of such hemorrhages are small, flamed-shaped lesions radiating from the optic disc and are parallel and superficial to the vessels. The incidence of hemorrhage varies with the

Table 5.17. Incidence of Retinal Hemorrhage in Spontaneous and Instrumental Delivery, Selected Series

Author	Delivery Type and % Retinal Hemorrhage[a]				
	Spontaneous (%)	Forceps (%)	Vacuum (%)	Cesarean (%)	N
Giles (64)	34	45			100
Ibanez et al. (65)	34	31	59	4	435
Krebs & Jager (66)	20		41		550
Krauer-Mayer (67)	20	19	50		212
Sezen (68)	14	33	40	1	1238
Ehlers et al. (69)	28	38	64		413
Zisa et al. (70)	11	27	30	2	1095
Besio et al. (71)	38	25		3	71
Levin et al. (72)	39	29	44	12	410
Egge et al. (73)	41	16	50		200
Mean percentage	27	29	42[b]	2[b]	4724

[a]Rounded to nearest whole percent.
[b]$P < 0.05$.

period of time from birth as well as the skill with which the ophthalmoscopic examination is performed. Most retinal lesions resorb within 24–48 hours. For example, in examination of 1238 newborns, Sezen observed a relatively low incidence of retinal hemorrhage (18.9%) at 24 hours (68). But between the third and fifth day this number rapidly dropped until by the fifth day in only 2.6% of his initial group of neonates could hemorrhages still be observed (68). Giles (64) observed a similar progressive disappearance of retinal lesions when serial examinations were performed on 100 neonates during the first 72 hours of life (Table 5.18). It can be theorized that hemorrhages result from unequal orbital or possibly cranial pressure distribution during birth, or the sudden release of extracranial pressure, dependent upon the rapidity and control of delivery of the fetal head.

There is a poor correlation between the incidence of retinal hemorrhage, maternal age, and parity. No correlation apparently exists between sex of the newborn, birth weight, or mean Apgar scores and the likelihood of hemorrhage. Cord complications, such as true knot or cord around the neck that are mentioned in older literature, also ap-

Table 5.18. Relationship between Time from Birth and Percentage of Retinal Hemorrhages Observed[a]

Hours after Delivery	Retinal Hemorrhages Observed in 100 Newborns[b] (%)
1	40
24	36
48	25
72	20

[a]From Giles CL. Retinal hemorrhages in the newborn. Am J Ophthalmol 1960; 49:1005–1011, published with permission from The American Journal of Ophthalmology. Copyright by The Ophthalmic Publishing Company, 1 December 1987.
[b]Full-term, examinations by direct ophthalmoscopy.

pear unrelated. Further, the incidence of retinal hemorrhage is apparently not significantly influenced by the concomitant use of electronic fetal monitoring during labor or oxytocin for induction or stimulation. Nor does hemorrhage seem to be influenced by the type of obstetric anesthesia or analgesia administered (72). However, there are positive associations between retinal hemorrhage, assisted delivery, and prolonged labor. *The most significant factor effecting incidence is mode of delivery.*

A number of studies are available in the literature on the incidence of retinal hemorrhage with spontaneous or assisted delivery, but these series vary in the period of time from birth, methods of examination, and how the hemorrhages are described (14, 67, 73). It is striking that hemorrhages are common, occurring in nearly one of three spontaneous and in an equal number of forceps-assisted deliveries. Cesarean section, in avoiding the second stage of labor or at least in avoiding vaginal expulsion and resultant fetal compression, is protective. Further, the incidence of retinal hemorrhage is lower in women in whom the duration of the first stage of labor is 1 hour or less and apparently in breech deliveries. Suggestions for the etiology of retinal hemorrhages include high pressure in the cavernous sinus, generalized increased intracranial pressure, fetal asphyxia/hypoxia, disorders of blood coagulation, and/or vitamin K deficiency, depression of the infant as indicated by the Apgar score, sex, cephalic molding, stress of the first breathing, and obstetrical trauma (64, 68, 71, 73). In general, retinal hemorrhage is probably related to changing pressure within the fetal cranium during the birth process (64, 73). The low incidence with cesarean delivery indicates that something about the molding and passage of the fetal head through the birth canal predisposes to the lesion. Management of the birth of the fetal head can also be important. Giles attended 100 full-term deliveries and subsequently examined the fundi of the resulting neonates (64). He felt that spontaneous deliveries with "poor head control" predisposed to retinal hemorrhage and reported an incidence of 70% in this subgroup although the numbers involved were small. These data suggested to him that with the infant's passage through the birth canal intracranial venous congestion occurred, which was released with delivery of the head. For example, increased venous pressure in the cavernous sinus can increase ophthalmic venous congestion. Thus, Giles argued, changes in pressure were dependent upon the management of the expulsion of the fetal head. With well-controlled delivery of the head, the pressure fluctuation would not be abrupt, and presumably the incidence of hemorrhages is less.

There are other data to review on considering the etiology of retinal hemorrhage. Inconsistent data suggest a higher incidence of hemorrhages in nulliparous women (73, 74). However, when the mode of delivery is factored in as a variable, the difference of parity disappears. This indicates that the actual methods of delivery are of greater importance than parity in the determining the total number and severity of retinal hemorrhages.

There is general agreement that there is a higher incidence of hemorrhages after delivery by vacuum extraction (73, 74). Further, the type of hemorrhage following vacuum extraction differs from that following spontaneous or forceps-assisted delivery. Why vacuum extraction has a particularly high incidence of lesions is unclear. The hypothesis of Egge et al. (73) is that vacuum extraction causes a temporary impairment of blood flow in the cavernous sinus and the bridging veins leading to venous stasis and resultant retinal bleeding. The apparent protective effect of outlet forceps may be to dampen pressure fluctuations within the fetal head by what Egge and coworkers called a "helmet" effect. Severe retinal hemorrhages—especially bleeds larger than the size of the optic disc and/or combined with periretinal hemorrhages—occur five times more frequently in neonates delivered by vacuum extraction than among those delivered either spontaneously or by forceps. There are data from the vacuum extraction literature indicating that the *location* of the vacuum extractor cup can effect the incidence of hemorrhage, but the numbers are too small to be consequential (67, 72). The period that vacuum is applied is also important. The longer the extraction, the greater the incidence of hemorrhages (74). In sum, it is clear that the majority of hemorrhages occur as a result of some type of spontaneous or induced obstetrical trauma but the definitive mechanism for these disorders is not established (64).

Retinal hemorrhages are classified based on the shape and size. As mentioned earlier, the smaller, irregular, and superficial hemorrhages disappear rapidly, usually within 72 hours. Round, redder, deeper hemorrhages are not as numerous and disappear over a longer time period, usually requiring 14–21 days or longer. The larger hemorrhages tend to occur more frequently when vacuum extraction has been used (67). Classifications of hemorrhages according to morphology have been numerous. However, the clinical significance seems to have more connection with the rate of disappearance, likely corresponding to a localization in or in front of the retina.

The clinical significance of retinal hemorrhage is not established but most data suggest that these lesions are transient events related to the birth process, leaving no lasting ill effects. The best information to date (72) fails to find any correlation between the ocular findings at birth and later childhood visual development.

Other eye injuries at delivery can be severe. Descemet's membrane can be ruptured by misapplication of forceps. The mechanism of damage by forceps is apparently compression of the globe against the superior orbit by the forceps blade slipping over the inferior orbital wall. Excessive horizontal stretching causes vertically oriented ruptures (75). This lesion can mimic the defect in Descement's membrane seen in congential glaucoma (16). If the damage is extensive, corneal edema, photophobia and tearing may also occur, further confusing the distinction between the traumatic lesion and true congenital glaucoma. Ophthalmologic evaluation by an experienced examiner is required to establish the correct diagnosis if a newborn is suspected of having a traumatic eye injury. This disorder has the potential for permanent injury. In seven cases followed for up to 60 years, when Descemet's membrane rupture occurred at birth associated with forceps delivery, marked astigmatism and myopia in the involved eye were present in all the individuals examined (75).

Rarely, hyphemas and vitreous hemorrhages accompany ruptures of Descemet's membrane. Hyphema usually resolves spontaneously. Vitreous hemorrhage is more serious and the prognosis guarded. If spontaneous resolution of a vitreous hemorrhage does not occur within 6–12 months, surgical exploration should be considered (16).

Intracranial Hemorrhage/Injury

Diagnosis. The clinical presentation on instrumental injury is variable. Drowsiness, pallor, poor cry or feeding, unexplained dyspnea or cyanosis, poor muscule tone, convulsions, or emesis can be noted. A history of difficult labor/delivery or birth asphyxia is common. The presence of cephalhematomas, lacerations, extensive ecchymoses, or fractures may accompany the more serious occult injury.

Incidence. Schenker and Serr (30) estimate an incidence of approximately 1.5% in cases involving instrumental delivery.

Comments. Intracranial hemorrhage is a serious complication of delivery and is associated with a likelihood of fetal death. Knowledge of basic newborn cranial anatomy is essential to an understanding of trauma-related intracranial bleeding. The intracranial compartments of the brain of the newborn/fetus are separated vertically by the falx cerebri and horizontally by the leaves of the tentorium cerebelli (Fig. 5.2) (21, 22). These structures consist of firm connective tissues. The falx is usually thinner than the tentorium and normally includes anterior fenestrations of varying sizes. The leaves of the falx and tentorium consist of two-layered radiating fibers, strengthened

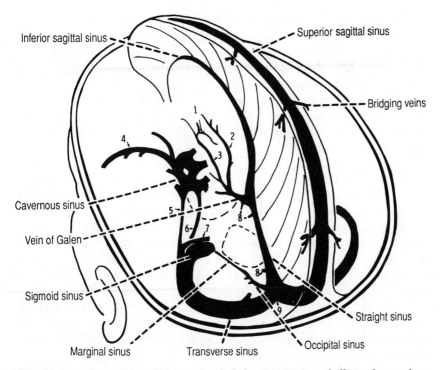

Figure 5.2.   Anatomy of the falx cerebri and the tenorium cerebelli in the newborn brain. Intracranial venous sinuses include: *1*, terminal vein; *2*, basal vein; *3*, internal cerebral vein; *4*, sphenoparietal sinus; *5*, superior petrosal sinus; *6*, inferior petrosal sinus; *7*, petrosal vein of Dandy; *8*, superior cerebellar veins; *9*, torcular herophili. (From Pape WE, Wigglesworth JS. Haemorrhage, Ischaemia and the Perinatal Brain. Philadelphia: JB Lippincott, 1979.)

with additional bands of fibers at the free margins. These tissue planes are accompanied by thin-walled venous sinuses which are particularly susceptible to traumatic injury (22). Under normal circumstances, the fetal head withstands molding and compression without difficultly. Simply put, damage to the falx and/or venous sinuses results from excessive frontooccipital compression or various forms of oblique distortion resulting from spontaneously occurring or induced cranial deformation. Cranial distortion results in kinking or obstruction of the vein of Galen or the related superior cerebellar veins. Oblique compression is caused by lateral force on the head—for example as might occur during the incorrect forceps application. This places one tentorium leaf under tension while relaxing the opposite one. This results in uneven transcranial pressure and predisposes to rupture of one of the bridging veins by stretching the connective tissues beyond the limits of their normal elasticity (76). The usual site of subdural

hemorrhage is the superior cerebellar bridging veins. Tentorium ruptures commonly involve the free margin close to the junction with the
falx. Rarely such tears may extend immediately into the straight sinus
or into the lateral sinus. Hemorrhage into the posterior fossa is an
important cause of death with cranial trauma. Damage to the superior
cerebellar veins and the straight and occipital sinuses is often the
source of such hemorrhages. The latter are at risk in cases involving
fracture/dislocation in the occipital region as described under "Skull
and Facial Fractures."

Skull and Facial Fractures

Diagnosis.   Skull fractures are identified either by direct observation or following radiographic studies. Such injuries are commonly accompanied by soft tissue injury or cephalhematoma. Skull
fractures may be either linear or of the depressed or ping-pong ball
type (77). Radiographic studies are indicated if extensive cephalhematomas are noted—especially bilateral hematomas—or other evidence of major cranial trauma is present (37). Usually the infant's ac-
tivity/behavior is normal unless concomitant hemorrhage is present. In
the uncommon event of basal skull fracture, drainage of bloody cer-
ebrospinal fluid from ears or nose, shock, or variable neurologic abnormalities can also be present.

Incidence.   The actual incidence is uncertain but such lesions
are uncommon. Spontaneously occurring, depressed fractures have
been described in sporadic case reports with and without instrumental
delivery (77). Linear fractures occur rarely in precipitous, spontaneous
deliveries. Cooke (4) reported an incidence of 0.475% for fractures observed when midpelvic rotational forceps deliveries were performed.

Comments.   The fetal skull is capable of considerable cranial
distortion without fracture. The fetal skull bones are poorly mineral-
ized and easily deformed. Further, the cranial bones are separated into
plates which are flexible between the suture lines, permitting considerable motion. The most common nondepressed fracture at postmortem examination is linear fracture of the parietal bone, usually
extending radially along the lines of cleavage. Such linear fractures
occur in association with cephalhematomas. Kendall and Woloshin
(78) described this association in 25% of their cephalhematoma series.
However, Zelson and Coworkers (37) noted a much lower incidence
(5.4%) of fracture with hematoma, unless the cephalhematoma was
bilateral (18% incidence), implying greater cranial trauma. Such fractures are uncommonly of clinical significance, although they may be
accompanied by extradural hemorrhages which can be serious. Depressed or "ping-pong ball" fractures are common and virtually al-

ways of the frontal and parietal bones but they are apparently of little serious consequence as long as promptly elevated and concomitant extradural hemorrhages are excluded (79). Of interest, slow spontaneous elevation may occur without neurological difficulties in smaller lesions and surgical intervention may not always be required (80). Such depressed fractures can be elevated by vacuum, as with a breast pump (81). It is possible but uncommon for depressed fractures to occur in utero. Such lesions are either associated with fetal skull impingement on the promontory of the sacrum or are from accidental trauma to the maternal abdomen. Rarely, leptomeningeal cysts develop from fracture sites (82, 83). The cyst is formed when an arachnoid herniation protrudes through a dural laceration present as a scalp mass. Fluid can then collect under the arachnoid, widening the cranial defect. The mass can be pulsatile and transilluminate. The cyst can increase in size with time, widening the cranial defect. There is invariably underlying brain injury. These cysts are commonly associated with seizures and should be surgically excised.

Occipital bone injuries deserve special consideration. Separation of the squamous and lateral portions of the occipital bone (occipital osteodiastasis) is a potentially serious condition and occasionally proves fatal (21). Excessive pressure on the suboccipital region during parturition results in traumatic separation of the cartilaginous joints between the segments of the bone. The lower edge of the squamous occipital bone is displaced and rotated forward toward the spinal canal. This is accompanied by dural and occipital sinus lacerations, gross subdural hemorrhage and, occasionally, laceration of the cerebellum. The most common abnormality is, however, not hemorrhage but displacement, compressing the posterior fossa. The extent of compression is variable and the lesion is by no means always fatal. As with the majority of spinal trauma this injury occurs most commonly following vaginal breech delivery. However, it has also been described in at least one instance following Kielland forceps rotation for a transverse arrest (21).

As long as epidural hemorrhage is absent, most skull fractures are not of great clinical consequence and complete recovery is the rule. However, the presence of the fracture implies traumatic delivery and/or the use of excessive force. Basal skull fractures are a different matter. These lesions are serious and carry a poor prognosis. If separation of the basal and squamous portions of the occipital bone occurs, either the outcome is fatal or serious neurological sequelae are found in survivors (14). When major scalp lesions or other evidence of cranial trauma are present after delivery, skull radiographs are prudent.

The most common facial fractures associated with delivery involve the nasal septum. The injury is usually a dislocation or fracture of the nasal bones and/or septum and occurs predominately in persisting occiput posterior presentations. In cases of nasal fracture/dislocation, respiratory embarrassment and/or neonatal feeding problems can result. According to Jeppesen and Windfeld (84) 3.2% of all deliveries are associated with dislocation of the nasal septal cartilage. There is an association between such injuries, nulliparity, prolonged second stage of labor, forceps applications, and certain obstetrical procedures such as the Mauriceau-Smellie-Veit maneuver. Such injuries are rarely, if ever, of clinical consequence.

Rarely the mandible is also fractured during the birth process (85). Early reduction and immobilization of mandibular fractures is desirable as rapid healing occurs.

Dentists and orthodontists have pointed out a possible relationship between malocclusion, mandibular hypoplasia, or other dental defects and a history of difficult instrumental delivery (86–90). An association between abnormalities of the mandible and instrumental delivery may not be as unlikely as it appears initially. The cartilage of the condylar process of the mandible is particularly vulnerable to trauma and genetic influences. Abnormalities can lead to unilateral or bilateral disturbances in growth. Injuries to the epiphysis of the mandible are reflected clinically as malformations or asymmetries in growth of the lower face or aberrant dental development. There is weak clinical evidence for the association of forceps delivery with malformations of teeth (87), asymmetric development of the mandible (86), and cross-bite abnormalities (88). Unfortunately, these studies are a blend of case reports and speculation with little solid data. Some retrospective data are more interesting but still flawed. Clayman and Goldberg (89) compared 219 patients with temporal mandibular joint problems against a control series matched for race, sex, and age. These authors noted that 55.7% of the patients with temporomandibular joint (TMJ) problems had been delivered by forceps (unspecified) while in the control group the use of forceps was reportedly 9.3%. This study is flawed for a number of reasons including problems with retrospective record evaluation and inconsistencies in the control group. However, these data suggest that an association *can* exist.

Spinal Cord Injuries

Diagnosis. The majority of spinal cord lesions occur in the cervical cord (91). Absent or difficult respiration is the most common clinical sign. Flaccid paralysis of the lower extremities is also observed on closer inspection. Respiratory distress, intercostal paralysis, retracted thorax, and a prominent abdomen during diaphragmatically controlled inspiration is present. The extremities are usually atonic, areflexic, and flaccid. The bladder may not empty until overflow occurs. Brachial plexus injury or fractures may be present in instances of difficult breech delivery. Radiographs of the spine are usually normal. An examination of the cerebral spinal fluid reveals blood. The differential diagnosis includes asphyxia neonatorum, intracranial injury, transverse myelitis, spinal cord tumors, spinal dysplasia and amyotonia congenita (92).

Incidence. A spinal cord injury incidence of 0.3% for midforceps with rotation is reported by Dunlop (2). The incidence following breech presentation is low unless undiagnosed hyperextension of the fetal head is present.

Comments. The spinal cord is fixed to the surrounding vertebral column and is not usually damaged during parturition unless unusual circumstances exist (91, 93). Despite presence of even complete cord transection, dislocation or fracture of the vertebral column is distinctly uncommon. While the cord itself is delicate and relatively inelastic, the bony vertebral column is quite easily stretched due to the relative weakness of the muscles and the elasticity of the connecting ligaments. Further, the spinal cord is tethered at both ends and capable of compression and/or direct injury. Thus, damage to the cord directly or to its supporting vascular structures commonly occurs without evidence of concomitant vertebral dislocation or fracture. Cord injury usually consists of a cervical or high thoracic cord lesion, including partial or complete laceration. Dural tears, avulsion of the cervical nerve roots, and spinal epidural hemorrhage can also occur. As noted, approximately 75% of the lesions result from difficult breech delivery but spinal cord lesions are also uncommonly seen during cephalic presentations and following midpelvic forceps rotations (92, 94). Spinal injuries associated with breech delivery are thought to be due to excessive longitudinal stretching of the fetal body, hyperextension of the head, ischemic injury due to narrowing or occlusion of vertebral arteries, or excessive nerve traction via the brachial plexus. Similar injuries rarely occur with spontaneous cephalic delivery and in association with shoulder dystocia (Table 5.19).

In the late 19th century, experiments on fresh stillborn fetuses were performed (99). By simulating footling breech extraction with the progressive application of weight, it was observed that spinal column rupture occurred consistently between cord segments C4 and C7. Direct linear force similar to that mimicked in these studies is likely related to cases of spinal injury in difficult version and extraction—procedures now passé. The mechanism is likely different in instances of cord injury associated with hyperextension of the fetal head during breech delivery—so-called "star gazing" or "flying fetus." It is postulated that acute angulation/hyperextension of the fetal head occurs just

Table 5.19. Spinal Cord Injuries, Cephalic Presentation Delivery[a]

Author	N	Delivery Details	Comments
Spencer[b]	6		Stillborns, spinal cord hemorrhage
Jolly[b]	1	Forceps rotation with conversion of face to vertex presentation (instrument unspecified)	Symmetrical arm paralysis, diagnosis presumptive
Couvelaire[b]	4		Dystocia present, hemorrhage into medulla and upper spine
Stoltzenberg[b]	1		Neonatal death from "ruptured spinal column"
Belfrage[b]	1	Spontaneous delivery, occiput posterior	Lesion at T_2
Crothers & Putnam[b]	4	"Difficult" forceps, second twin, one high, others unspecified, one shoulder dystocia	Cervical cord injuries, one scapular fracture, accompanying brachial plexus injury in four
	3	Spontaneous deliveries, one shoulder dystocia	
Föderl[b]	1		High cervical cord lesion, with subluxation of cervical spine
Herzog[b]	1	Spontaneous delivery	Lesion at T_{10}, scoliosis and spastic paraplegia
Towbin (91)	2[c]	One spontaneous (?)	5120 g intrapartum death, C_4-T_3 epidural hemorrhage
		One high forceps	Cerebellar contusion and cord hemorrhage
Walter & Tedeschi (95)	2	33 weeks, 760 g, chronic membrane rupture	Probable oligohydramnios, IUGR[d],
		35.5 weeks, 2835 g uncomplicated delivery respiratory distress	Epidural and subdural hemorrhage
Shulman et al. (96)	1	Midpelvic rotation, occiput posterior to occiput anterior (instrument unspecified)	Lesion at C_1-C_2 and spinal fracture/ dislocation, general anesthesia for delivery
Pridmore (97)	1	Midpelvic rotation, right occiput posterior to occiput anterior (Kielland)	Marked oligohydramnios, general anesthesia for delivery, lesion at C_2
Pape and Wigglesworth (22)	1	Midpelvic rotation (Kielland)	"Difficult" delivery, transection of medulla, occipital osteodiastasis and tentorial tear
Gould and Smith (98)	1	Midpelvic rotation, left occiput anterior to occiput anterior, fetal distress (Kielland)	Lesion at C_2-C_3, no bony injury or dural tears

[a]Modified from Shulman ST, Madden JD, Esterly JR, Shanklin, DR. Transection of spinal cord: a rare obstetrical complication of cephalic delivery. Arch Dis Child 1971; 46:291–294.
[b]Quoted by Shulman.
[c]Report indicates two possible additional cases apparently involving spinal epidural hemorrhage, details scanty.
[d]IUGR, intrauterine growth retardation.

prior to flexion during the delivery process as the fetal body is delivered. The nonossified segments of the newborn's cervical vertebrae permit greater latitude of motion than is possible in the adult spinal column, resulting in compression and shearing forces which compromise the blood supply or effectively pinch the cervical cord. Thereafter, hemorrhage and edema result in physiologic cord transection.

The best treatment is prevention. Avoidance of breech extraction in singleton presentations and great care and routine use of Piper forceps during elective term breech delivery reduces the risk (100, 101). As noted, in very rare instances, midpelvic rotational forceps deliveries can also result in spinal column damage. The presumed mechanism is forceful traction plus angulation of the vertebral column. The true incidence of cervical lesion during midpelvic rotational deliveries cannot be accurately estimated as it occurs sporadically and is rare. It is not clear what constellation of circumstances are required to produce such damage (Table 5.19).

Treatment is supportive and often unsatisfactory. Infection, fecal retention, and problems with skin breakdown are common. Prognosis is dependent upon the severity of the lesion, the quality of supportive care, and whether infection becomes a serious problem. Many neonates with serious spinal injury die in infancy, commonly of ascending urinary tract infection.

Fractures (Clavicle, Humerus, Femur)

Diagnosis. At birth, with some green-stick and most complete fractures, arm movement is reduced or absent. Dislocation or obvious deformity may be present. Passive movement usually elicits cries of pain from the infant. Palpation reveals tenderness, swelling, or irregularity. Radiographs confirm the diagnosis (14).

Incidence. The incidence of fracture is generally low and in most series less than 1% (Table 5.20).

Table 5.20. Incidence of Clavicular and Humerus Fractures with Operative Delivery, Selected Series

Author	Delivery Type	Incidence (%)	Comments
Clavicle			
Widen et al. (31)	Unspecified	0.02	
Dunlop (2)	Midforceps with rotation	0.3	Forceps, type unspecified
Hughey et al. (50)	Midforceps with rotation	0.7	Forceps, type unspecified
Gilstrap et al. (7)	Low forceps	0.2	Forceps, type unspecified
Benkus et al. (34)	Vacuum extraction cases	1.2	
Humerus			
Hughey et al. (50)	Midforceps with rotation	0.2	Forceps, type unspecified

Comments. The clavicle is the most commonly fractured bone during birth. The fracture usually occurs during delivery of a macrosomic or breech infant. Undisplaced fractures require no specific therapy beyond immobilization of the arm and shoulder to minimize pain. Displaced fractures are immobilized with a figure eight bandage to prevent potential injury to either the brachial plexus or the apex of the pleural cavity. Rarely is surgical exploration required and recovery is usually rapid and complete. On occasion, fracture of the clavicle produces a pseudo-Erb's palsy, in which the neonate does not use a limb, and nerve injury to the brachial plexus is suspected. An area of obvious induration or tenderness, usually in the midportion of the clavicle, will be noticed on careful examination.

The most common long bone fractures are those of the humerus and femur. Three-quarters of birth-associated fractures of the long bones occur in breech presentation. The majority of the remainder occur with shoulder dystocia. Fractures of the humerus usually occur in the middle third of the shaft and are either transverse or spiral. These may be associated with transient radial nerve injury. In cephalic presentations the humerus can be fractured by traction, particularly while disengaging an impacted shoulder or arm during shoulder girdle dystocia. Femoral shaft fractures usually occur in the middle third of the bone and are usually transverse. The injury is normally caused by traction on the legs during breech delivery. Traumatic separation of the upper femoral or humeral epiphysis can occur in either setting outlined above which may mimic dislocation or fracture.

Facial Nerve Palsy

Diagnosis. When nerve injury occurs, decreased or absent movements of the eyelid, lip, and facial muscles are observed in the distribution of the VII (facial) cranial nerve. Commonly, the deficit is unilateral, and facial asymmetry is present, particularly during facial grimacing or spontaneous crying. When the child cries, the eyeball rolls up but the lid remains open. Touching the cornea does not evoke any local lid response but the eyeball will roll upward and the *opposite* lid will close. In complete lesions, drooping or sagging of the affected cheek and mouth edge is present (102).

Incidence. The incidence of VII nerve palsy in noninstrumented deliveries is difficult to estimate. The disorder does occur spontaneously due to compression of the nerve trunk or its fibers before or during parturition. Rubin (24) observed 21 cases in 15,435 births (0.14%), 19 of these (90%) associated with forceps. McHugh et al. noted 41 injuries in 18,139 consecutive births (0.25%) (102). In contrast, Hepner reported an incidence of 6.3% in 159 spontaneous labors (103). In modern series, the overall incidence approximates 0.5/ 1000 livebirths (104, 105). The reported incidence of facial palsy in series of forceps deliveries varies greatly—from 0.1 to 12% (Table 5.21). As the injury results in a deficit which is striking to attendants and parents, it is unlikely that the diagnosis is overlooked when significant nerve trauma occurs. Sampling problems and differences in the incidence of instrumental delivery likely explain the wide range in reported incidence.

VIIth nerve palsies are associated with forceps use, duration of the second stage of labor, nulliparity, and fetal size greater than 3500 g (20). The disorder is much more common when vaginal delivery has occurred. Sharma et al. (106), for example, observed no instances following cesarean section. However, as the numbers in this study were 100 and the incidence of the disorder so low, it cannot be concluded that cesarean delivery is invariably protective. Hepner (103) reported two instances following cesarean section in women with platypelloid pelves where the facial paresis occurred on the same side of the fetal head as the occiput prior to delivery. Further, in the series of Smith et al. (104) 9 of the 74 cases of facial weakness occurred in deliveries in which forceps had not been used.

There remains some uncertainty about the role of forceps in producing facial nerve palsy. Hepner (103) observed that the incidence of facial nerve palsy was virtually identical among 716 infants delivered with the use of forceps versus 159 without forceps (6.4 versus 6.3%). However, data from other series support the belief that facial palsy is more common among infants delivered with forceps assistance. In cases unassociated with forceps, it is probable that pressure from the maternal sacral promontory or possibly the infant's own shoulder is the cause of injury (103, 107). Of interest, Hepner's study (103) revealed a consistent association between the position of the fetal head and the side of facial paresis. For example, his series included 46

Table 5.21. Reported Incidence of Facial Palsy following Forceps Delivery

Author	Type of Forceps Delivery	%
Hepner (103)	Unspecified	6.4
Rubin (24)	Unspecified	0.12
Shenker & Serr (30)	Unspecified	0.3
Sharma et al. (106)	Unspecified	12.0
Cooke (4)	Mid	4.2
Dunlop (2)	Mid, no rotation	0.7
Smith et al. (104)	Manual rotation and forceps	2.0
Healy et al. (32)	Mid with Rotation	1.3
Hughey et al. (50)	Mid with Rotation (non-Kielland)	2.0
Healy et al. (32)	Kielland	1.0

infants with facial paresis who had undergone forceps delivery. Thirty-four had left facial paresis and all were described as presenting in left occiput to anterior position. The remaining 12 newborns had right facial paresis. All were born from right occiput positions.

Comments. Traumatic nerve injury must be differentiated from developmental anomalies of the facial nerves, muscles, or central nerve nucleus (105, 108). Excluding trauma, the most common abnormalities affecting facial nerve function are the Möbius syndrome and congenital absence of the depressor anguli oris muscle. In general, developmental anomalies associated with facial palsy are associated with anomalies of the face or ear, other cranial nerve abnormalities (nerves III, IV, V, IX, X, and XII), partial defects in facial functions, radiographic abnormalities of the temporal bone, abnormalities in brainstem auditory evoked responses and include a family history of the same defect (108). Some children have other associated congenital anomalies involving the cardiovascular, skeletal, or genitourinary systems (109). In differentiating traumatic from developmental palsies, electrophysiologic testing can be helpful. When a developmental abnormality is the cause, facial nerve conduction studies are usually immediately abnormal at birth. In contrast, with traumatic injuries, nerve conduction studies are usually normal and become abnormal only several days after the injury (105). If the axon is severed, wallerian degeneration occurs. This is reflected by 3–7 days of age by progressive reduction in the amplitude of the evoked compound motor unit potential. Later, by 10–14 days, fibrillation potentials or other abnormal spontaneous activity potentials are observed (105).

Injury is due to direct pressure on the VIIth nerve, although the source of pressure and the mechanism for its application are controversial. The nerve is more superficial and slightly higher in its course in newborns than in adults (102, 110). At birth neither the mastoid bone nor the stylomastoid process are fully developed and do not entirely shield the VIIth nerve as it exits from its foramen (102, 110). In the skull of the newborn, the facial nerve emerges directly from the stylomastoid foramen onto the lateral surface of the skull, covered initially only by the posterior digastric muscle and the overlying sternomastoic muscle insertion. Rarely the nerve is injured due to basilar skull fracture that entraps the nerve in its bony canal. Hemotypanum is an important clinical sign of possible fracture (111). The nerve can also be compressed in its more peripheral branches. This is felt to occur due to the observation that in some cases not all segments of the nerve are equally involved (111). Apparently the VIIth nerve can also be injured if the overlying temporal bone is indented but not fractured during delivery by compressing or crushing the nerve in the canal (105).

If the lesion occurs, spontaneous recovery for 90% is the rule and commonly occurs within the first month, although delayed recovery is possible (105, 112). A rapid recovery is virtually assured unless there is a central lesion. In a difficult case the clinician must exclude other causes of apparent VIIth nerve palsy including congential abnormalities in the nerve nucleus (Möbius syndrome) or muscles of facial expression (16, 104, 108). Surgery for VIIth nerve lesions needs to be approached conservatively in most instances (105). First, the majority of injuries spontaneously resolve without therapy. Second, there are no controlled studies demonstrating an improved outcome for surgical explanation/decompression of the nerve. Finally, surgical exploration can result in further nerve injury. However, some neonates are candidates for exploration (113, 105). Bergman et al. (105) suggest surgical exploration be considered if unilateral and complete paralysis is present at birth, if there is a displaced fracture of the petrous bone and hemotympanum, or if electrophysiologic studies demonstrate absence of voluntary *and* evoked motor unit responses in all muscles innervated by the facial nerve by 3–5 days of life or if there is no return of function clinically or electrophysiologically by 5 weeks of age. Apparently neonates with traumatic facial palsy, even with poor prognostic signs, can still make a rapid and complete spontaneous recovery. Thus, to minimize the necessity for unnecessary exploration without a reduction in the likelihood for long-term repair, observation for up to 5 weeks is indicated. Even if spontaneous improvement does not occur, the delay neither substantially reduces the likelihood for surgical repair nor leads to additional nerve damage. Management consists of reassurance to the parents and protecting the corneal epithelium if inadequate closure of the eye is present. Electrodiagnostic testing should be performed in establishing a correct diagnosis. Further, all such infants should undergo careful clinical assessment to judge the extent of the defect. An otoscopic examination for hemotympanum is indicated, as is observation for periaural ecchymosis (104) to help exclude skull fracture/hematoma. Other supportive measures include facial muscle massage and controlled electrostimulation of the nerve, where intact (113). In selected cases, surgical exploration and/or nerve reconstruction is rarely required.

Rare Complications

Among the rarest of complications associated with instrumental delivery is brain tissue embolization during delivery. Brain tissue embolization has been reported in adults and children as a rare complication of cranial injury (114–116). Of 7 cases reported in neonates and reviewed by Wannakrairot and Shuangshoti (117), 4 were associated with breech presentation and forceps use. All 7 newborns died within 1 hour of delivery. There is some evidence suggesting that embolization can be associated with long-term survival. Pulmonary nodules of neural tissue thought to result from remote traumatic injuries have been described, although in 5 of 6 cases severe brain abnormalities were also present (116). It is presumed that these instances represent cases in which fragments of neural tissue, previously embolized, survive in an ectopic locale. It can be theorized that brain tissue is forced into open venous channels during the birth process. Reversal of flow in cerebral flow due to changing pressures on the great vein of Galen presumably results in systemic embolization (114, 116, 118). A potential clinical problem of direct embolization of brain tissue is activation of the coagulation cascade due to the brain's high thromboplastic activity (119, 120).

Soft tissue injuries to the ear are also occasionally seen in association with forceps delivery. The incidence of significant trauma is surprisingly small, with the vast majority of lesions of no clinical consequence. Ecchymoses, abrasions, and very uncommonly lacerations and hematomas may be observed. Incision and drainage of hematomas may be necessary. Lacerations are repaired with 5-0 suture material. If the cartilage is involved, particular care is necessary and expert consultation is required (14).

Mortality

The ultimate and feared complication of any obstetric procedure is death. As the accompanying table (Table 5.22) indicates, series reporting forceps deliveries vary substantially in the number of infant deaths associated with forceps use. Most infant deaths associated with forceps applications are due to intracranial hemorrhages or fractures of the skull with or without accompanying spinal cord lesions (Table 5.23). The majority of these injuries occur in more difficult forceps applications but can be seen rarely even in apparently easy procedures. The wide range of incidence reflects both the care with which unexplained stillborns or neonatal deaths are subjected to careful anatomic necropsy as well as the original indications for forceps application.

Complications of Vacuum Extraction

Vacuum extraction, like all forms of instrumental delivery, is associated with maternal and fetal complications (Table 5.24). Fortunately, most are minor. Uncommonly, as with forceps, major maternal/fetal complications of vacuum extraction do occur and some can prove

Table 5.22. Infant Death Associated with Forceps Delivery, Selected Series

Reference	N	%	Comments
Kielland forceps: midforceps			
Chiswick & James (121)	86	3.4	All tentorial tears
Burke & Wood (122)	75	0	
Healy et al. (32)	552	1.27	
Unspecified forceps type; midforceps with rotation			
Hughey et al. (50)	458	0.7	
Healy et al. (32)	95	1.05	
Unspecified forceps type; midforceps, rotation included			
Decker et al. (123)	547	3.1	
Cosgrove & Weaver (6)	1,000	1.2	
Midforceps without rotation			
Steer (124)		4	
Taylor et al. (3)	31	26	
Kirk et al. (125)	254	0	
Cooke (4)	427	0	Mostly DeWees' forceps
Dunlop (2)	292	0	
Friedman (126)		1.89	
Low forceps			
Friedman (126)		0.6	
Parallel blade forceps			
Seidenschmur & Koepcke (127)	1,503	0.19	Shute forceps, two tentorial tears, one traumatic subdural and subarachnoid hemorrhages
Shute (128)	2,092	0.09	One depressed skull fracture, one compressed and lacerated cord
Unspecified forceps procedures			
Nyirjesy et al. (129)	29,186	0	

quite serious. All neonates subjected to vacuum extraction will have ecchymoses and a chignon of some extent at the site of the vacuum cup attachment. This swelling varies with the type of extraction device used and is most marked when the rigid or semirigid cups have been used. Such abnormalities are transient and generally of cosmetic interest only. This is not to say that such lesions are inconsequential. The intitial striking appearance of the chignon and the occasional associated cephalhematomata are a major reason why vacuum extraction has never gained great popularity in the United States.

Maternal Complications

The most common maternal injury associated with vacuum extraction is episiotomy extension. Traction in the pelvic curve and the necessity to apply force as nearly perpendicular to the vacuum cup face as possible means that episiotomy is often required. Close attention to detail in repair with particular care to note occult fourth degree

Table 5.23. Neonatal Mortality—Case Reports

Reference	Cause	Comments
Towbin (91)	Contusion and fragmentation of cerebellum	High forceps applied, slipped, and reapplied
Schulman et al. (96)	Transection spinal cord	Term, cephalic presentation, occiput posterior with rotation by midforceps
Norman & Wedderburn (130)	Spinal cord damage, two case reports	Cephalic, left occiput posterior midforceps, slight shoulder dystocia Cephalic, right occiput transverse, manual rotation
Gariepy & Fugere (120)	Pulmonary embolization of cerebellar tissue	Piper forceps, breech presentation
Pridmore et al. (97)	Cervical cord laceration	Kielland forceps, lesion probably due to rotation rather than traction
Gould & Smith (98)	Spinal cord transection	Kielland forceps, rotation from left occiput anterior
O'Driscoll et al. (131)	IVH[a]	27 cases

[a]IVH, intraventricular hemorrhage.

(rectal) extensions is required. Secondary breakdown of such lacerations/extensions and formation of fistulae is uncommon and infection surprisingly infrequent. Such episiotomy extensions have the same clinical import as those associated with forceps.

If careful attention is not given to the cup margin when vacuum is applied, redundant maternal tissues may be trapped and lacerated. Either the lateral vaginal wall or the cervix can be injured. On occasion, visualization of blood in the vacuum tubing or in the suction trap will alert the clinician. As in all instrumental deliveries, a close

Table 5.24. Complications Associated with Vacuum Extraction

Maternal
  Lacerations: cervix, lateral vaginal walls, extension of episiotomy
  Fistula formation (vesicovaginal, rectovaginal)
Fetal
  Shoulder girdle dystocia, Erb/Duchenne palsy
  Scalp injury: lacerations, abrasions, ecchymoses, necrosis, infection, anemia, hyperbilirubinemia
  Cephalhematoma
  Subgaleal (subaponeurotic) hematoma
  Skull fracture, disruption of sutures
  Intracranial hemorrhage
  Retinal hemorrhage

inspection of the birth canal upon completing a vacuum-assisted delivery is mandatory. The best treatment for these maternal injuries is prevention, with rigid adherence to the protocol for vacuum extractor application.

Fetal Complications

Damages to the infant from vacuum extraction are predominately those of scalp injury and retinal hemorrhage. Intracranial injuries also occur, but these are rare. Perinatal mortality in collected series averages 15.5/1000 (Table 5.25).

Shoulder Girdle Dystocia, Erb/Duchenne Palsy

Comments. There is apparently an increase in shoulder dystocia with midpelvic vacuum extractions (155). The extractor does not

Table 5.25. Perinatal Mortality in Vacuum Extraction (VE) Deliveries[a]

Series	No. of VE Deliveries	Deaths	Perinatal Mortality p/1000 VEs	Corrected Perinatal Mortality x/1000 VEs[b]
Evelbauer (132)	580	6	NR[c]	10
Holtorff (133)	119	2	17	8
Berggren (134)	100	6	60	20
Zilliacus & Sjöstedt (135)	508	10	NR	20
Brandstrup & Lange (136)	651	28	43	NR
Grossard & Cohn (137)	92	1	10.9	0
Hammerstein & Gromotke (138)	365	3	NR	7
Aguero & Alvarez (139)	100	5	50	NR
Porpakkham (140)	652	40	109	59
Brey et al. (141)	213	7	33	NR
Roszkowski et al. (142)	521	7	13.4	NR
Malmström (143)	520	12	23	10
Lasbrey et al. (144)	121	2	18	NR
Eggers et al. (145)	102	4	37.5	20
Chalmers (146)	700	5	7	NR
Brat (147)	1135	41	36.3	19.4
Barth & Newton (148)	100	3	30	0
Popa et al. (149)	550	10	18	NR
Schenker & Serr (30)	299	5	16	12
Widen et al. (31)	201	6	30	NR
Matheson et al. (150)	168	3	18	NR
Chalmers & Prakash (151)	201	3	15	NR
Bjerre & Dahlin (152)	101	2	19.6	NR
Plauché (153)	228	4	19	NR
Total	8327	215	25.8	15.5[c]

[a]Modified from Plauché WC. Fetal cranial injuries related to delivery with a Malmström vacuum extractor. Obstet Gynecol 1979; 53:750–757.
[b]x, perinatal deaths not attributable to the extractor.
[c]NR, not reported.

increase the size of the mass to be delivered and can be more easily applied than forceps. Thus, macrosomic infants, who might have failed forceps application or have been considered as candidates for a trial, can be delivered by vacuum extraction. Please refer to the discussion in the previous section concerning forceps operations.

Scalp Injury: Lacerations, Abrasions, Ecchymoses, Necrosis, Infection, Anemia, Hyperbilirubinemia

Diagnosis.   Scalp injury is diagnosed by direct observation of the vacuum site on the neonatal scalp.

Incidence.   Plauché (154) in his review of 3543 vacuum extractions using the Malmström cup calculates a mean incidence of minor scalp trauma of 12.6% (Table 5.26). The series vary greatly in how these lesions were diagnosed or reported.

Comments.   All experienced users of vacuum extraction appear to concur that minor scalp abrasions and ecchymoses are common, but of little clinical importance. At times such lesions are of substantial cosmetic consequence. Significant scalp injuries are often due to operator inexperience, especially failure to follow guidelines for the period of time for allowable vacuum and avoidance of cup detachment, especially when the rigid metal extractors are used. In general, no treatment is necessary for ecchymoses as long as the infant's skin remains intact. If a raw or denuded area develops, careful cleansing with surgical soap and the use of a topical antibiotic oint-

Table 5.26.   Abrasion and/or Laceration of Fetal Scalp in Vacuum Extractor (VE) Deliveries[a]

Series	No. of VE Deliveries	No. of Scalp Abrasions or Lacerations	%
Mishell & Kelly (156)	25	4	16.0
Grossard & Cohn (137)	92	6	6.52
Munsat et al. (157)	109	13	11.9
Guardino & O'Brien (158)	114	1	0.8
Roszkowski et al. (142)	521	196	37.6
Malmström (143)	520	89	17.1 (superficial)
Barth & Newton (148)	100	3	3.0
St. Vincent Buss (159)	199	25	12.5
Brat (147)	1135	10	0.88
Schenker & Serr (30)	299	15	5.0
Chalmers & Prakash (151)	201	66	33.0 (minor)
Plauché (153)	228	19	8.4
Broekhuizen et al. (160)	256	113	44.1 (minor)
Total	3799	560	Mean 14.7

[a]Reprinted with permission from The American College of Obstetricians and Gynecologists (From Plauché WC. Fetal cranial injuries related to delivery with a Malmström vacuum extractor. Obstet Gynecol 1979; 53:750–757).

ment is appropriate. Extensive scalp injuries must be carefully evaluated to exclude underlying skull fractures, hematomas, or other lesions (Fig. 5.3).

Cephalhematomas

Diagnosis. A cephalhematoma consists of a collection of blood under the scalp in a newborn infant (Fig. 5.1). The lesion results from an effusion of fetal blood beneath the pericranium due to laceration of subperiosteal vessels. Cephalhematomas develop when a shearing displacement of the soft tissues of the scalp occurs as they are displaced to and fro over the more rigid underlying bone during spontaneous or instrumentally assisted delivery (161). Cephalhematomas are to be contrasted with caput succedaneum and subaponeurotic hemorrhages. In caput succedaneum, the effusion is entirely independent of the periosteum of the bone and consists of serum. In cephalhematomas, the swelling is contained by suture line which usually sharply delimits the lesion. Clinically, large cephalhematomas may be

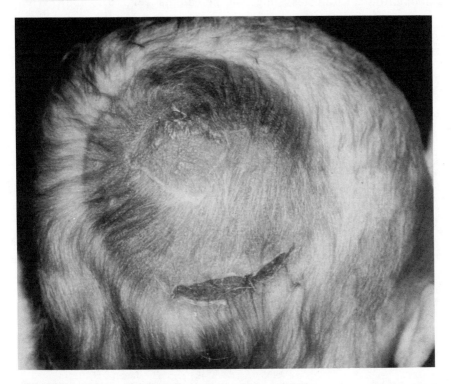

Figure 5.3.   Scalp ecchymosis following prolonged metal-cup vacuum extraction (Bird modification).

difficult to distinguish from caput succedaneum (see prior section on forceps injuries).

Incidence. Cephalhematomas occur significantly more frequently in instrumental deliveries than in spontaneous delivery, especially with midforceps and vacuum extraction (Table 5.27).

Comment. Cephalhematomas may be large and misdiagnosed as scalp edema (caput succedaneum). Occasionally, neonatal anemia or hyperbilirubinemia results from the hemorrhage and its subsequent resorption (165). Such lesions are common with vacuum extraction but usually minor, resolving spontaneously without specific therapy. The vast majority are of no clinical consequence.

Skull Fracture

(See discussion under "Forceps Operations.")

Subgaleal (Subaponeurotic) Hematoma

Diagnosis. A collection of blood in the potential space between the periosteum of the skull (paracranium) and the galea aponeurotica indicates subgaleal hematoma (Fig. 5.1) (38). When

Table 5.27. Cephalhematomata in Vacuum Extraction (VE) Deliveries[a]

Series	No. of VE Deliveries	No. of Cephalhematomata	%
Amosy & Ahlander (162)	216	5	2.3
Zilliacus & Sjöstedt (135)	508	40	7.9
Brandstrup & Lange (136)	651	36	5.5
Mishell & Kelly (156)	25	2	8.0
Spritzer (163)	60	3	4.2
Hammerstein & Gromotke (138)	365	18	4.9
Guardino & O'Brien (158)	114	7	6.1
Munsat et al. (157)	109	28	25.9
Roszkowski et al. (142)	521	31	5.95
Lasbrey et al. (144)	121	20	17.0 ("often small")
Malmström (143)	520	68	13.2
Barth & Newton (148)	100	18	18.0
Chalmers (146)	700	7	1.0 (+4.5% scalp effusion)
St. Vincent Buss (159)	199	11	5.5
Brat (147)	1135	27	2.4
Schenker & Serr (30)	299	12	4.0
Widen et al. (31)	201	11	5.5
Fahmy (164)	2670	117	4.4
Plauché (153)	228	23	10.0
Boekhuizen et al. (160)	256	10	3.9
Total	8998	494	Mean 5.5%

[a]Modified from Plauché WC. Fetal cranial injuries related to delivery with a Malmström vacuum extractor. Obstet Gynecol 1979; 53:750–757.

subaponeurotic hemorrhage occurs, diffuse swelling of the scalp is observed, which can be indented with finger pressure (166). The hematoma may also present as a fluid swelling indistinguishable from scalp edema, commonly situated over the occipital region. Scalp discoloration from blood extravasation can appear in the frontal or occipital regions of the newborn's head. Uncommonly with large hemorrhages, the entire scalp is tense to palpation. Especially if the disorder occurs rapidly, hypotension and palor may be the only signs. A rising pulse rate, increased respiratory rate, and possibly a documentation of a rapid drop in hemoglobin/hematocrit in an infant with scalp lesions suggest the correct diagnosis. As the disorder progresses, signs of cerebral irritation may occur and convulsions ensue (38, 166–170).

Incidence.   It is difficult to determine the spontaneous incidence of subgaleal hemorrhage. Plauché estimated the overall incidence to be 4/10,000 deliveries (38). The condition is uncommon and is unusual after spontaneous vaginal delivery. However, it is difficult to tease out a rate related to vacuum extraction or to forceps delivery. The disorder may be underreported or reported under alternative names. As can be seen from Table 5.28, the lesion has been reported either rarely (171, 172) or commonly (166) in cases of vacuum extraction. In Plauché's 1980 review of 123 cases, approximately one-half occurred after vacuum extraction and one-third during spontaneous vaginal delivery. The best estimate of overall risk approximates 1% in vacuum-extracted infants.

Comments.   Subgaleal hematomas are potentially serious and differ from cephalhematomas. Cephalhematomas are collections of blood beneath the periosteum and are confined in size by the limits of a single cranial bone due to the firm attachments of the periosteum at the periphery of each bony plate. However, subgaleal hemorrhage is outside the periosteum, beneath the galea, and thus can extend across suture lines (see Fig. 5.1). Large quantities of blood can collect rapidly,

Table 5.28. Incidence of Subgaleal Hemorrhage (Subaponeurotic Hemorrhage) Following Vacuum Extraction[a]

Author	No. of Vacuum Extractions	No. of Hemorrhages	%
Malmström (143)	520	2[b]	0.38
Lange (171)	922	3	0.32
Ahuja et al. (166)	310	13[c]	4.2
Chalmers (172)	1500	15	1.0
Total	3252	33	1.0%

[a]Modified from Plauché WC. Fetal cranial injuries related to delivery with a Malmström vacuum extractor. Obstet Gynecol 1979; 53:750–757.
[b]Two cases required transfusion.
[c]3/13, 23.1% proved fatal. 6/13 cases resulted when forceps application followed vacuum extraction.

especially if any concomitant abnormality in coagulation is present (166). In his study of 310 infants delivered by vacuum extraction, Ahuja showed that subaponeurotic or galeal hemorrhage was significantly more frequent when vitamin K-dependent coagulation factors (factors II, IV, VII, and X) were at low levels (166). Administration of parenteral vitamin K to the neonate has little effect on preventing this disorder as the increase in coagulation activity is not rapid enough to offset the hemorrhage. Clinically, the hemorrhage may appear as soon as 1½ hours or as late as 48 hours after birth. In nonfatal cases the retained hemoglobin can give rise to hyperbilirubinemia and neonatal jaundice (165). There are a number of reports which indicate that this disorder is more common in males and in neonates of African and non-Caucasian origin. (38, 166, 168–170) The volume of blood loss in subgaleal hemorrhage is often underestimated and vigorous support is necessary. The treatment is transfusion of fresh whole blood and cardiovascular support. Fresh frozen plasma and vitamin K_1 (phytonadione) can also be given and application of pressure bandages to the fetal head can be considered. In the review of Plauché, 28 of 123 neonates with subgaleal hematomas died, for a mortality rate of 22.8% (38).

Intracranial Hemorrhage/Signs of Cerebral Irritation

Incidence.   In collected series the incidence varies from 0.2 to 8% (Table 5.29). The overall incidence is approximately 0.75%. Long-term follow-up studies have observed few residual deficits (Table 5.30).

Diagnosis.   The most common presentation is neonatal depression, apnea, or shock. Occasionally increased irritability or poor feeding is observed. Fits or convulsions occur occasionally. The diagnosis is suspected especially when abnormal neonatal behavior accompanies clinical evidence of cranial injury.

Comments.   There is clinical evidence that elective vacuum extraction does not cause fetal hypoxia (182). While difficult vacuum extractions commonly produce scalp injuries, serious cranial damage is rare (172). Intracranial hemorrhage has been reported after vacuum extraction delivery. However, the indications for the procedure and technique play a prominent part in the occurrence of trauma and there is evidence that preexisting hypoxia increases the risk of intracranial damage (183).

Newer techniques have been used to investigate the cranium of newborns subjected to vacuum extraction. Computerized axial tomography has not found a good correlation between the incidence of intracranial hemorrhage and the mode of delivery, although such anal-

Table 5.29. Intracranial Hemorrhage (ICH) in Vacuum Extraction (VE) Deliveries[a]

Author	No. of VE Deliveries	No. of ICH Cases	% ICH
Bruniquel & Dollar (173)	148	2	1.4
Lacomme et al. (174)	60	2	3.3
Chalmers & Fothergill (175)	100	1	1.0
Bergman & Malmström (176)	1617	2	0.2
Aguero & Alvarez (139)	100	8	8.0
Roszkowski et al. (142)	521	4	0.77
Lange (177)	922	7	0.76
Amosy & Ahlander (162)	216	1	0.46
Lasbrey et al. (144)	121	1	0.8
Bergman & Malmström (176)	520	3	0.58
Chalmers (146)	700	6	0.87
Brat (147)	1135	1	0.08
Schenker & Serr (30)	299	2	0.6
Bjerre & Dahlin (152)	101	1	1.0
Porpakkham (140)	652	10 (5 had forceps after VE)	1.53
Total	7124	52	Mean 0.72 (0.35 entire series)

[a]Many series report no cases of intracranial bleeding. Total number of VEs reviewed was 14,276. Modified from Plauché WC. Fetal cranial injuries related to delivery with a Malmström vacuum extractor. Obstet Gynecol 1979; 53:750–757.

Table 5.30. Long-term Neurologic Damage of Infant after Vacuum Extraction (VE) Deliveries[a]

Series	No. of Cases	Controls	Duration of Follow-up	CNS Damage[b] VE (%)	Controls (%)
Malmström & Jansson (178)	520	120	To 10 years	"No reason to change positive attitude toward VE"	
Eggers et al. (145)	102		1–3½ years	7 slight 9 marked	
Popa et al. (149)	327		1–3 years	0	
Earn (179)	100		1–6 years	0	
Brandstrup & Lange (136)	651		To 10 years	0	
Brey et al. (141)	63		1 year	16	
Bjerre & Dahlin (152)	101	120	4 years	5.3	5.9
Bliennow et al. (180)	40		14 months	0[c]	
Meyer et al. (181)	380		3–11 years	17 mild 6.1 marked	10 mild 3.7 marked

[a]Reprinted with permission from The American College of Obstetricians and Gynecologists (From Plauché WC. Fetal cranial injuries related to delivery with a Malmström vacuum extractor. Obstet Gynecol 1979; 53:750–757).
[b]CNS, central nervous system.
[c]Nine infants with "behavioral problems": colic (6), disturbed sleep (5), breath-holding spells (2), unusual sound insensitivity (3).

Table 5.31.   Clinical Signs of Neurologic Damage of Newborn after Delivery: Vacuum Extraction (VE) versus Forceps[a]

	VE		Forceps		Spontaneous	
	Range	Mean %	Range	Mean %	Range	Mean %
Retinal hemorrhage	20–66	44	28–31	30	14.6–33.6	22.6
Cerebral irritation	0.1–5.1	3.3	2.7–4	3.4		
Abnormal EEG	7–59	29		44.6[b]	5.5–13.7	9.6

[a]Reprinted with permission from The American College of Obstetricians and Gynecologists (From Plauché WC. Fetal cranial injuries related to delivery with a Malmström vaccum extractor. Obstet Gynecol 1979; 53:750–757).
[b]Mean range only reported in one study.

yses are at best controversial. Ultrasound has also been used for similar evaluations. While limited data are available for vacuum extraction infants, a study of 28 neonates by Jeannin et al. (182) failed to find any evidence of intracranial hemorrhage or subdural effusions in patients studied 72 hours after delivery. Five of the 28 infants had fetal heart rate bradycardias as an indication for assisted delivery and the other applications were elective or indicated for a delay in the second stage. In four instances, scalp abrasion was noted and in five cases a cephalhematoma was observed. Awon (184) has described the distortion of the fetal parietal bone when vacuum extraction is applied to the fetal head. It is theorized that such distortion might lead to disruption of intracranial vessels and to hemorrhage. However, there is some controversy about Awon's finding as his studies were performed on fresh stillborns. Whether the distortions depicted in his radiographs are reflective of what occurs in the intact and living fetus is controversial. When clinical signs of neurologic damage (retinal hemorrhage, cerebral irritation, abnormal EEG) are compared between instrumental and spontaneous delivery, there is in general a higher incidence of these disorders whenever instrumentation has occurred (Table 5.31). The incidence of cerebral irritation following both vacuum extraction and forceps application appears relatively similar except that retinal hemorrhages are more common in vacuum-extracted neonates, albeit of uncertain long-term implication.

Retinal Hemorrhage

(See discussion under "Forceps Operations.")

REFERENCES

1. Simpson JY. Societies. In: Speert H, ed. Obstetrics and gynecology in America: a history. Baltimore: Waverly Press, 1980:118.

2. Dunlop DL. Midforceps operations at the University of Alberta Hospital (1965–1967). Am J Obstet Gynecol 1969; 103:471–475.

3. Taylor E. Can mid-forceps operations be eliminated? Obstet Gynecol 1953; 2:302–307.
4. Cooke WAR. Evaluation of the midforceps operation. Am J Obstet Gynecol 1967; 99:327–332.
5. Danforth DN, Ellis AH. Midforceps delivery—a vanishing art? Am J Obstet Gynecol 1963; 86:29–37.
6. Cosgrove RA, Weaver OS. An analysis of 1,000 consecutive midforceps operations. Am J Obstet Gynecol 1957; 73:556–558.
7. Gilstrap LC, Hauth JC, Schiano S, Conner KD. Neonatal acidosis and method of delivery. Obstet Gynecol 1984; 63:681–685.
8. Borkowf HI. Bacterial gangrene associated with pelvic surgery. Clin Obstet Gynecol 1973; 16:40–65.
9. Shy KK, Eschenbach DA. Fatal perineal cellulitis from an episiotomy site. Obstet Gynecol 1979; 54:292–298.
10. Rea WJ, Wyrick WJ. Necrotizing fasciitis. Ann Surg 1970; 172:957–964.
11. Janevicius RV, Hann S-E, Batt MD. Necrotizing fasciitis. Surg Gynecol Obstet 1982; 154:97–102.
12. Meleney FL. Hemolytic streptococcus gangrene. Arch Surg 1924; 9:317–364.
13. Meleney FL. Hemolytic streptococcus gangrene: importance of early diagnosis in an early operation. JAMA 1929; 92:2009–2012.
14. Margurten HH. Birth injuries in neonatal-perinatal medicine. 4th ed, St Louis: Mosby, 1987.
15. Gresham EL. Birth trauma. Pediatr Clin North Am 1975; 22:317–328.
16. Curran JS. Birth-associated injury. Clin Perinatol 1981; 8:111–129.
17. Illingworth RS. A paediatrician asks—why is it called birth injury? Br J Obstet Gynaecol 1985; 92:122–130.
18. Joshi VV. Primary causes of perinatal mortality: autopsy study of 100 cases. Arch Pathol Lab Med 1976; 100:106–109.
19. Valdes-Dapena MA, Arey JB. The causes of neonatal mortality: an analysis of 501 autopsies on newborn infants. J Pediatr 1970; 77:366–375.
20. Levine MG, Holroyde J, Woods JR, Siddiqui TA, MacHenry S, Mi-
odovnik M. Birth trauma: incidence and predisposing factors. Obstet Gynecol 1984; 63:792–795.
21. Wigglesworth JS. Perinatal pathology. Philadelphia: WB Saunders, 1984.
22. Pape WE, Wigglesworth JS. Haemorrhage, Ischaemia and the Perinatal Brain. Philadelphia: JB Lippincott, 1979.
23. Madsen ET. Fractures of the extremities in the newborn. Acta Obstet Gynecol Scand 1955; 34:41–74.
24. Rubin A. Birth injuries: incidence, mechanisms, and end results. Obstet Gynecol 1964; 23:218–221.
25. Tan KL. Brachial palsy. J Obstet Gynaecol Br Commonw 1973; 80:60–62.
26. Gordon M, Rich H, Deutschberger J, Green M. The immediate and long-term outcome of obstetric birth trauma. I. Brachial plexus paralysis. Am J Obstet Gynecol 1973; 117:51–56.
27. Cohen AW, Otto SR. Obstetric clavicular fractures: a three-year analysis. J Reprod Med 1980; 25:119–122.
28. Munsat TL, Neerhout R, Nyirjesy Y. A comparative clinical study of the vacuum extractor and forceps. Part II. Evaluation of the newborn. Am J Obstet Gynecol 1963; 85:1083–1090.
29. Churchill JA, Stevenson L, Habhab G. Cephalhematoma and natal brain injury. Obstet Gynecol 1966; 27:580–584.
30. Schenker JG, Serr DM. Comparative study of delivery by vacuum extractor and forceps. Am J Obstet Gynecol 1967; 98:32–39.
31. Widen JA, Erez S, Steer CM. An evaluation of the vacuum extractor in a series of 201 cases. Am J Obstet Gynecol 1967; 98:24–31.
32. Healy DL, Quinn, MA, Pepperell RJ. Rotational delivery of the fetus: Kielland's forceps and two other methods compared. Br J Obstet Gynaecol 1982; 89:501–506.
33. Vacca W, Grant A, Wyatt G, Chalmers I. Portsmouth operative delivery trial: a comparison vacuum extraction and forceps delivery. Br J Obstet Gynaecol 1983; 90:1107–1112.
34. Benkus MD, Ramamurthy RS,

O'Connor PS, Brown K, Hayashi RH. Cohort studies of silastic obstetric vacuum cup deliveries: I. Safety of the instrument. Obstet Gynecol 1985; 66:503–509.

35. Yasunaga S, Rivera R. Cephalhematoma in the newborn. Observations based on a review of 139 infants. Clin Pediatr 1974; 13:256–260.

36. Bresnan MJ. Neurologic birth injuries. Part I. Postgrad Med 1971; 49:191–205.

37. Zelson C, Lee SJ, Pearl M. The incidence of skull fractures underlying cephalhematomas in newborn infants. J Pediatr 1974; 85:371–373.

38. Plauché WC. Subgaleal hematoma: a complication of instrumental delivery. JAMA 1980; 244:1597–1598.

39. Mazzanti GA. Delivery of the anterior shoulder. Obstet Gynecol 1959; 13:603–607.

40. Schramm M. Impacted shoulders—a personal experience. Aust NZ J Obstet Gynaecol 1983; 23:28–31.

41. Benedetti TJ, Gabbe SG. Shoulder dystocia. A complication of fetal macrosomia and prolonged second stage of labor with midpelvic delivery. Obstet Gynecol 1978; 52:526–529.

42. Benedetti TJ. Managing shoulder dystocia. Contemp Obstet Gynecol 1979; 14:33–40.

43. Woods CE. A principle of physics as applicable to shoulder delivery. Am J Obstet Gynecol 1943; 45:796–804.

44. Resnik R. Management of shoulder girdle dystocia. Clin Obstet Gynecol 1980; 23:559–564.

45. Schwartz BC, Dixon D. Shoulder dystocia. Obstet Gynecol 1958; 11:468–471.

46. Seigworth GR. Shoulder dystocia: review of 5 years experience. Obstet Gynecol 1966; 28:764–767.

47. McFarland LV, Raskin M, Daling FR, Benedetti TJ. Erbs/Duchenne's palsy: a consequence of fetal macrosomia and method of delivery. Obstet Gynecol 1986; 68:784–788.

48. Swartz DP. Shoulder girdle dystocia in vertex delivery: clinical study and review. Obstet Gynecol 1960; 15:194–206.

49. McCall JO. Shoulder dystocia: A study of after effects. Am J Obstet Gynecol 1962; 83:1486–1490.

50. Hughey MJ, McElin TW, Lussky R. Forceps operations and perspective. I. Midforceps rotation operations. J Reprod Med 1978; 20:253–259.

51. Gebbie D. Symphysiotomy. Clin Obstet Gynecol 1982; 9:663–683.

52. Sandberg EC. The Zavanelli maneuver: a potentially revolutionary method for the resolution of shoulder dystocia. Am J Obstet Gynecol 1985; 152:479–484.

53. Pearse WH, Danforth DN. Dystocia due to abnormal fetopelvic relations. In: Danforth DN, Dignam WJ, Hendricks CH, Maeck JUS, eds. Obstetrics and gynecology. 3rd ed. Hagerstown, Maryland: Harper & Row, 1977: 628–647.

54. Hibbard LT. Shoulder dystocia. Obstet Gynecol 1969; 34:424–429.

55. Gonik B, Stringer CA, Held B. An alternate maneuver for management of shoulder dystocia. Am J Obstet Gynecol 1983; 145:882–884.

56. Shute WB. Management of shoulder dystocia with the Shute parallel forceps. Am J Obstet Gynecol 1962; 84:936–939.

57. Hadlock FP, Harrist RB, Sharman RS, Deter RL, Park SK. Estimation of fetal weight with the use of head, body and femur measurements—a prospective study. Am J Obstet Gynecol 1985; 151:333–337.

58. Boyd ME, Usher RH, McLean FH. Fetal macrosomia: prediction, risks, proposed management. Obstet Gynecol 1983; 61:715–722.

59. Williams J, Kirz DS, Worthen NJ, Oakes GK. Ultrasound prediction of shoulder dystocia [Abstract 11]. Society of Perinatal Obstetricians Annual Meeting, Fifth Annual Clinical Scientific and Business Meeting, 31 January–2 February, 1985: 27.

60. Eng GD. Brachial plexus palsy in newborn infants. Pediatrics 1971; 48:18–28.

61. Vassalos E, Prevedourakis C, Paraschopoulou-Prevedouraki P. Brachial plexus paralysis in the newborn. Am J Obstet Gynecol 1968; 101:554–556.

62. Specht EE. Brachial plexus palsy in the newborn: incidence and prognosis. Clin Orthop Relat Res 1975; 110:32–34.

63. Chen TH, Shewmake SW, Hansen DD, Lacey HL. Subcutaneous fat necrosis of the newborn. Arch Dermatol 1981; 117:36.

64. Giles CL. Retinal hemorrhages in the newborn. Am J Ophthalmol 1960; 49:1005–1011.

65. Ibanez JMS, Gonzalez NB, Martinez AN. Retina-hämorrhagien beim neugeborenen nach vakuum-extraktion. Gynaecol 1963; 156:172–186.

66. Krebs W, Jager G. Retinal hemorrhage in newborn infants and the course of delivery. Klin Monatsbl Augenheilkd 1966; 148:483–490.

67. Krauer-Mayer B. Sur les hemorragies retiniennes du nouveau-né: une étude comparative après accouchement spontané, par extracteur pneumatique ou par forceps. Gynecol Obstet (Paris) 1966; 65:77–82.

68. Sezen F. Retinal hemorrhages in newborn infants. Br J Ophthalmol 1970; 55:248–253.

69. Ehlers N, Jensen IK, Hansen KB. Retinal haemorrhages in the newborn: comparison of delivery by forceps and by vacuum extractor. Acta Ophthalmol (Copenk) 1974; 52:73–82.

70. Zisa F, Capozzi A, Ceccarello PL. Incidencza delle lesioni vascolari retiniche conseguenti al parto. Minerva Ginecol 1975; 27:294–297.

71. Besio R, Caballero C, Meerhoff E, Schwarcz R. Neonatal retinal hemorrhages and influence of perinatal factors. Am J Ophthalmol 1979; 87:74–76.

72. Levin S, Ganive J, Mintz M, Kreisler C, Romem M, Klutznik A, Feingold M, Insler V. Diagnostic and prognostic value of retinal hemorrhages in the neonate. Obstet Gynecol 1980; 55:309–314.

73. Egge K, Lyng G, Maltau JM. Effect of instrumental delivery on the frequency and severity of retinal hemorrhages in the newborn. Acta Obstet Gynecol Scand 1981; 60:153–155.

74. Schenker JG, Gombos GM. Retinal hemorrhage in the newborn. Obstet Gynecol 1966; 27:521–524.

75. Angell LK, Robb RM, Berson FG. Visual prognosis in patients with ruptures in Descemet's membrane due to forceps injuries. Arch Ophthalmol 1981; 99:2137–2139.

76. Courville CB. Birth and brain damage. Pasadena, Church Press, 1971: 25.

77. Axton JHM. Depressions of the skull in the newborn. Nurs Mirror 1966; 4:123–124.

78. Kendall N, Woloshin H. Cephalhematoma associated with fracture of the skull. J Pediatr 1952; 41:125–132.

79. Harwood-Nash DC, Hendrick EB, Hudson AR. The significance of skull fractures in children. Radiology 1971; 101:151–155.

80. Loesser JP, Kilburn HL, Jolley T. Management of depressed skull fracture in the newborn. J Neurosurg 1976; 44:62–64.

81. Schragen GO. Elevation of depressed skull fracture with a breast pump. J Pediatr 1970; 77:300–301.

82. Kingsley D, Till K, Hoare R. Growing fractures of the skull. J Neurol Neurosurg Psychiatry 1978; 41:312.

83. Genieser NB, Becker MH. Head trauma in children. Radiol Clin North Am 1974; 12:333–342.

84. Jeppesen F, Windfeld I. Dislocation of the nasal septal cartilage in the newborn: aetiology, spontaneous course and treatment. Acta Obstet Gynaecol Scand 1972; 51:5–15.

85. Monks FT. A fractured mandible in the new-born. Br J Oral Surg 1977; 14:270–274.

86. Berger SS, Stewart RE. Mandibular hypoplasia secondary to perinatal trauma. J Oral Surg 1977; 35:578–582.

87. Bier-Katz VG. Traumatische schadigung eines bleibenden zahnes durch eine zangengeburt-eine fallbeschreibung. Dtsch Zahnaerztl Z 1975; 30:451–456.

88. Schoenwetter RF. A possible relationship between certain malocclusions and difficult or instrument deliveries. Angle Orthod 1974; 44:336–340.

89. Clayman GL, Goldberg JS. The incidence of forceps delivery among patients with TMJ problems. J Craniomandib Pract 1983; 2:46–50.
90. Via WF, Churchill JA. Relationship of enamel hypoplasia to abnormal events of gestation and birth. J Am Dent Assoc 1959; 59:702–707.
91. Towbin A. Spinal cord and brain stem injury at birth. Arch Pathol 1964; 77:620–632.
92. Stern WE, Rand RW. Birth injuries to the spinal cord: a report of 2 cases and review of the literature. Am J Obstet Gynecol 1959; 78:498–512.
93. Towbin A. Central nervous system damage in the human fetus and newborn infant. Am J Dis Child 1970; 119:529–542.
94. Crothers B, Putnam MC. Obstetrical injuries of the spinal cord. Medicine (Baltimore) 1927; 6:41–126.
95. Walter CE, Tedeschi LG. Spinal injury and neonatal death: report of six cases. Am J Obstet Gynecol 1970; 106:272–278.
96. Shulman ST, Madden JD, Esterly JR, Shanklin DR. Transection of spinal cord: a rare obstetrical complication of cephalic delivery. Arch Dis Child 1971; 46:291–294.
97. Pridmore BR, Hey EN, Aherne WA. Spinal cord injury of the fetus during delivery with Kielland's forceps. J Obstet Gynecol Br Commonw 1974; 81:168–172.
98. Gould SJ, Smith JF. Spinal cord transection, cerebral ischaemic and brain-stem injury in a baby following a Kielland's forceps rotation. Neuropathol Appl Neurobiol 1984; 10:151–158.
99. Dohrmann GJ. Experimental spinal cord trauma: a historical review. Arch Neurol 1972; 27:468–473.
100. Piper EB, Bachman C: The prevention of fetal injuries in breech delivery. JAMA 1929; 92:217–221.
101. Milner RDG. Neonatal mortality of breech deliveries with and without forceps to the aftercoming head. Br J Obstet Gynaecol 1975; 82:783–785.
102. McHugh HE, Sowden KA, Levitt MN. Facial paralysis and muscle agenesis in the newborn. Arch Otalaryngol 1969; 89:157–169.
103. Hepner WR. Some observations on

104. facial paresis in the newborn infant: etiology and incidence. Pediatrics 1951; 8:494–497.
104. Smith JD, Crumley RL, Harker LA. Facial paralysis in the newborn. Otolaryngol Head Neck Surg 1981; 89:1021–1024.
105. Bergman I, May M, Wessel HB, Stool SE. Management of facial palsy caused by birth trauma. Laryngoscope 1986; 94:381–384.
106. Sharma U, Idnani N, Saxena S. Effects of obstetrical interference on the newborn. Indian J Pediatr 1978; 45:143–153.
107. Parmelee AH. Molding due to intrauterine posture: facial paralysis probably due to such molding. Am J Dis Child 1931; 42:1155–1159.
108. Henderson JL. The congenital facial diplegia syndrome: clinical features, pathology and aetiology. Brain 1939; 62:381–403.
109. Pape KE, Pickering D. Asymmetric crying facies: an index of other congenital anomalies. J Pediatr 1972; 81:21–30.
110. Sammarco J, Ryan RF, Longenecker CG. Anatomy of the facial nerve in fetuses and stillborn infants. J Plastic Reconst Surg 1966; 37:556–574.
111. McLellan MS, Vautier T. Neonatal seventh nerve palsy in the absence of hemotympanum. Am J Obstet Gynecol 1973; 117:572–574.
112. Alberti PW, Biagioni E. Facial paralysis in children. A review of 150 cases. Laryngoscope 1972; 82:1013–1020.
113. Kornblut AD. Traumatic facial nerve injuries in children. Adv Otorhinolaryngol 1977; 22:171–181.
114. Tryfus H. Massive pulmonary embolism of cerebella tissue in a newborn. Arch Dis Child 1963; 38:292–294.
115. Levine, SB. Embolization of cerebral tissue to lungs. Arch Pathol 1973; 96:183–185.
116. Valdes-Dapena MA, Arey JB. Pulmonary emboli of cerebral origin in the newborn. Arch Pathol 1967; 84:643–646.
117. Wannakrairot P, Shuangshoti S. Cerebellar tissue embolism associated with birth injury. J Med Assoc Thai 1984; 67:290–294.
118. Gardiner WR. Massive pulmonary

embolization of the cerebeller cortical tissue: an unusual fetal birth injury. Stanford Med Bull 1956; 14:226–229.

119. Gagne F. Embolies pulmonaires de tissu cerebelleux chez le nouveau-né. Union Med Can 1970; 99:275–277.

120. Gariepy G, Fugere P. Pulmonary embolization of cerebellar tissue in a newborn child. Obstet Gynecol 1973; 42:118–120.

121. Chiswick ML, James DK. Kielland's forceps: association with neonatal morbidity and mortality. Br Med J 1979; 1:7–9.

122. Burke M, Wood C. Kielland's forceps. Letter to the editor. Br Med J 1979; 1:616.

123. Decker WH, Dickson WA, Heaton CE. An analysis of five hundred forty-seven midforceps operations. Am J Obstet Gynecol 1953; 65:294–303.

124. Steer CM. Effect of type of delivery on future childbearing. Am J Obstet Gynecol 1950; 60:395–400.

125. Kirk RF, Krumholz BA, Callagan Da. The mid-forceps operation. Prognosis based on pelvic capacity and fetal weight. Obstet Gynecol 1960; 15:447–451.

126. Friedman EA. Patterns of labor as indicators of risk. Clin Obstet Gynecol 1973; 16:172–183.

127. Seidenschnur G, Koepcke E. Fetal risk in delivery with the Shute parallel forceps. Am J Obstet Gynecol 1979; 135:312–317.

128. Shute WB. The parallel obstetrical forceps: reducing injuries during delivery. Med Trial Tech Q 1973; 19:272–282, 411–417.

129. Nyirjesy I, Hawks BL, Falls HC, Munsat TL, Pierce WE. A comparative clinical study of the vacuum extractor and forceps. Am J Obstet Gynecol 1964; 85:1071–1082.

130. Norman MG, Wedderburn LCW. Fetal spinal cord injury with cephalic delivery. Obstet Gynecol 1973; 42:355–358.

131. O'Driscoll K, Meager D, MacDonald D, Georghegan F. Traumatic intracranial haemorrhage in firstborn infants and delivery with obstetric forceps. Br J Obstet Gynaecol 1981; 88:577–581.

132. Evelbauer K. Experiences with the use of the vacuum extractor. Geburtshilfe Frauenheilkd 1956; 16:223.

133. Holtorff J. Infant mortality and morbidity in forceps and vacuum extraction. Zentralbl Gynakol 1961; 83:261–268.

134. Berggren OG. Experience with Malmström's vacuum extractor. Acta Obstet Gynecol Scand 1959; 38:315–332.

135. Zilliacus H, Sjöstedt E. Proceedings of the Third World Congress of the International Federation of Obstetrics and Gynecology, Vol I, Vienna: 1961:84.

136. Brandstrup E, Lange P. Clinical experience with the vacuum extractor. Proceedings of the Third World Congress of the International Federation of Obstetrics and Gynecology, 1961: 737.

137. Grossard P, Cohn S. The Malmström vacuum extractor in obstetrics. Obstet Gynecol 1962; 19:207–211.

138. Hammerstein J, Gromotke R. The value of Malmström's extractor in operative obstetrics. J Int Col Surg 1962; 37:458–462.

139. Aguero O, Alvarez H. Fetal injury due to the vacuum extractor. Obstet Gynecol 1962; 19:212–217.

140. Porpakkham S. Evaluation of the vacuum extractor used in the second stage of labor. Am J Obstet Gynecol 1962; 84:940–951.

141. Brey J, Holtorff J, Kintzel HW. Vacuum extraction with special reference to early and late infantile injuries. Geburtshilfe Frauenheilkd 1956; 22:550–560.

142. Roszkowski I, Borkowski R, Kretowicz J. Use of the vacuum extractor in fetal distress. Am J Obstet Gynecol 1963; 87:253–257.

143. Malmström T. The vacuum extractor. I. Indications and results. Acta Obstet Gynecol Scand 1964; 43(suppl):5–52.

144. Lasbrey AH, Orchard CD, Crichton D. A study of the relative merits and scope for vacuum extraction as opposed to forceps delivery. S Afr J Obstet Gynaecol 1964; 2:1–3.

145. Eggers H, Seidenschnur G, Wagner KD. Late clinical psychological, radiologic and electroencephalographic

findings after vacuum extraction. Geburtshilfe Frauenheilkd 1964; 24:295–301.

146. Chalmers JA. The vacuum extractor in difficult delivery. J Obstet Gynaecol Br Commonw 1965; 72:889–891.

147. Brat T. Indications for and results of the use of the "ventouse obstetricale" (a ten year study). J Obstet Gynaecol Br Commonw 1965; 72:883–888.

148. Barth WH, Newton M. The use of the vacuum extractor. Am J Obstet Gynecol 1965; 91:403–406.

149. Popa S, Herscu A, Stefant A. Vacuum extraction in the "Tudor Vladimiresch district maternity." Obstet Ginecol (Buchar) 1965; 13:503.

150. Matheson GW, Davajan V, Mishell DR. The use of the vacuum extractor, a reappraisal. Acta Obstet Gynecol Scand 1968; 47:155–165.

151. Chalmers JA, Prakash A. Vacuum extraction initated in the first stage of labour. J Obstet Gynaecol Br Commonw 1971; 78:554–558.

152. Bjerre I, Dahlin K. The long-term development of children delivered by vacuum extraction. Dev Med Child Neurol 1974; 16:378–380.

153. Plauché WC. Vacuum extraction. Use in a community hospital setting. Obstet Gynecol 1978; 52:289–293.

154. Plauché WC. Fetal cranial injuries related to delivery with a Malmström vacuum extractor. Obstet Gynecol 1979; 53:750–757.

155. McFarland LV, Raskin M, Daling JR, Benedetti TJ. Erb/Duchenne's palsy: consequence of fetal macrosomia and method of deliveries. Obstet Gynecol 1986; 68:784-788.

156. Mishell D, Kelly JV. The obstetrical forceps and the vacuum extractor: an assessment of their compressive force. Obstet Gynecol 1962; 19:204–206.

157. Munsat TL, Neerhout R, Jyirjesy I. A comparative clinical study of the vacuum extractor and forceps. Part II. Evaluation of the newborn. Am J Obstet Gynecol 1963; 85:1083–1090.

158. Guardino AN, O'Brien FB. Preliminary experiences with Malmström's vacuum extractor. Am J Obstet Gynecol 1962; 83:300–306.

159. St. Vincent Buss T. Vacuum extraction in the first stage of labor. S Afr J Obstet Gynaecol 1965; 3:53–57.

160. Broekhuizen FF, Washington JM, Johnson F, Hamilton PR. Vacuum extraction versus forceps delivery: indications and complications, 1979 to 1984. Obstet Gynecol 1981; 57:571–577.

161. Greenhill JP. Obstetrics. 3rd ed. Philadelphia: WB Saunders, 1965.

162. Amosy G., Ahlander K. Forceps delivery or vacuum extractor? A comparison over a five-year period. Nord Med 1960; 64:839–842.

163. Spritzer TD. Use of the vacuum extractor in obstetrics. Am J Obstet Gynecol 1962; 83:307–310.

164. Fahmy K. Cephalohaematoma following vacuum extraction. J Obstet Gynaecol Br Commonw 1971; 78:369–372.

165. Arad I, Fainmesser P, Birkenfeld A, Gulaiev B, Sadovsky E. Vacuum extraction and neonatal jaundice. J Perinat Med 1982; 10:274–278.

166. Ahuja GL, Willoughby MLN, Kerr MM, Hutchison JH. Massive subaponeurotic haemorrhage in infants born by vacuum extraction. Br Med J 1969; 3:743–749.

167. Andersson LO, Hansson G, Malmström T, Ryba W. Post-natal subgaleal haematomas. Acta Obstet Gynecol Scand 1963; 42:358–366.

168. Kumari S, Bhargava SK. Subaponeurotic haemorrhage in the newborn. J Indian Med Assoc 1977; 69:3–5.

169. Kagwa-Nyanzi JA, Alpidousky VK. Subaponeurotic hemorrhage in newborn infants: An analysis of nine instances in African infants. Clin Pediatr (Phila) 1972; 11:224–227.

170. Williams MF, Jacobs M, Moosa A. Subaponeurotic haemorrhage of the newborn. S. Afr Med J 1977; 52:176–178.

171. Lange P. The vacuum extractor: value in relation to forceps and range of indications. Acta Obstet Gynecol Scand 1964; 43(suppl):57–85.

172. Chalmers JA. The ventouse: the obstetric vacuum extractor. Chicago: Year Book, 1971.

173. Bruniquel G, Dollar H. Épreuve double aveugle sur les hemorragies retinennes du nouveau né: Resultats en contraction fornelle avec certaines

statistiques alarmantes après vacuum extractor. In: Hubinont P, Bradfer-Blomert J, Brat T, eds. Effects of vacuum extractor and a obstetrical forceps on the foetus and the newborn—comparison. Proceedings of the Fifth World Congress of Obstetrics and Gynecology, Sydney: September, 1967: 101–120.

174. Lacomme M, Lewin D, Thierry E. Forceps, spatules et ventouses. Rev Fr Gynecol Obstet 1965; 5:325–328.

175. Chalmers JA, Fothergill RJ. Use of a vacuum extractor (ventouse) in obstetrics. Br Med J 1960; 1:1684–1689.

176. Bergman P, Malmström T. Natal and postnatal foetal mortality in association with vacuum extraction and forceps delivery. Gynaecologia 1962; 154:65–72.

177. Lange P. Clinical experience with the vacuum extractor. Dan Med Bull 1961; 8:11–17.

178. Malmström T, Jansson I. Use of the vacuum extractor. Clin Obstet Gynecol 1965; 8:893–913.

179. Earn AA. An appraisal of Malmström's vacuum-tractor (vacuum extractor). Am J Obstet Gynecol 1967; 99:732–743.

180. Bliennow G, Svenningsen NW, Gustafson B, Sunden B, Cronquist S. Neonatal and prospective follow-up study of infants delivery by vacuum extraction (VE). Acta Obstet Gynecol Scand 1977; 56:189–194.

181. Meyer C, Geisert J, Durand de Bousingen R. Regarding neuropsychic residua of infants delivered by the Swedish ventouse. Rev Neuropsychiatr Infant Hyg Ment Enfance 1972; 20:343.

182. Jeannin P, Afschrift M, Voet F, Vandekerckhove F, Thiery M, Defoort P, Derom R. Cranial ultrasound after forceful midpelvis vacuum extraction at term. J Perinat Med 1984; 12:319–325.

183. Thiery M, VanKets H, Derom R. Recording of tractive power in vacuum extraction. J Perinat Med 1973; 1:291–292.

184. Awon MP. The vacuum extractor—experimental demonstration of distortion of the foetal skull. J Obstet Gynaecol Br Commonw 1964; 71:634–636.

6

Birth Events and Long-term Neonatal Disability

One has to consider that the anomaly of the birth process,
rather than being the causal etiologic factor, may itself be the
consequence of the real perinatal etiology.

SIGMUND FREUD, 1897 (1)

To those who concern themselves with the question of knowing
from the start if I have succeeded to the goal I have proposed,
I rely on the judgement of those who do not allow themselves
to be carried away by preconceived ancient opinions in
forming their own ...

F. ANTON MESMER, 1766 (2)

Introduction

There is no more controversial subject than the relationship between birth injuries and the long-term neonatal neurobehavioral disorders (3–13). This association is of great clinical importance. The rapid rise in cesarean delivery in the United States to approximately 20% is at least a partial reflection of the concern to avoid fetal trauma. The majority of cesarean sections are undertaken to avoid difficult delivery associated with dystocia, failure to progress, or malpresentation. No one practicing obstetrics in the United States is unaware of how such concerns color our handling of complicated cases. The constant threat of a bad result pervades our thinking and affects our management in subtle and nonsubtle ways. An example is the progressive decline in the teaching of breech delivery technique and/or in utero and extra utero manipulations for version for the delivery of the second twin. In both instances the data against vaginal delivery or intrauterine manipulations for term gestations are at best inconclusive. Yet, a climate of opinion has developed favoring abandonment of these classic obstetrical techniques/maneuvers. The effect(s) of such changes are long-term, with some results largely unforeseen. As fewer cases are performed, training lapses and eventually falls into abeyance as the ranks of skilled practitioners diminish. Eventually, the training of an entire generation of obstetricians is altered. To reverse such a trend is possible if a return to prior practice was desirable but the lag time is measured in years, independent of the issue of whether such changes in practice are indicated.

Similar issues concern instrumental delivery. It may or may not be appropriate for future obstetrical management to depend only upon outlet forceps/vacuum or cesarean section as companions to spontaneous delivery. In fact, this author thinks not. However, unless obstetric teaching of low forceps and midpelvic applications and the appropriate use of the vacuum extractor continues, within several years, markedly limited procedures will be all that many practitioners can safely perform.

Instrumental delivery is not without risk. It is clear that the more complex the instrumental intervention, the greater the likelihood of fetal and maternal damage. Midpelvic and rotational deliveries of more than 45° are associated with greater numbers of neonates with short- and long-term disability than is spontaneous delivery. Further, a larger proportion of neonates subjected to instrumental delivery will have depressed Apgar scores than those observed with spontaneous parturitions. But what do these associations mean? Is it the method of delivery alone that is responsible for the increased likelihood of a poor outcome? Does cesarean section conclude invariably with a better result? Can we estimate the risk to benefit ratio for instrumental delivery?

The Past as Prologue

As reviewed in Chapter 1, extreme attitudes concerning instrumental delivery have been common since the first use of forceps. In recent years a more critical view of instrumental delivery has emerged, leaving clinicians uncertain how to proceed and hesitant to use procedures in which they were originally trained. What is required is a balanced view of instrumental assistance in obstetrics with roles for forceps, vacuum extraction, and cesarean section. In this regard, a critical review of current data concerning ante- and intrapartum events and fetal/neonatal condition is in order.

Predictability of Developmental Abnormalities

Predicting eventual abnormal neonatal development from antenatal and intrapartum events is both complex and uncertain. There are associations between intrauterine asphyxia and poor long-term neonatal development (14, 15). Further, there is a common tendency to believe that there is a strong association between early fetal depression (as reflected primarily in the Apgar score) and neonatal complications; yet the evidence supporting the latter conclusion is at best limited (16). In fact, the evidence is *much* stronger that *antenatal* events are critical in many, if not most, cases of long-term neonatal neurodevelopmental morbidity (i.e., cerebral palsy) (12, 13, 15).

Asphyxia remains the major cause of perinatal morbidity and mortality (17). We cannot be certain that perinatal asphyxia is the *only* or even the major cause of cerebral palsy. Even under laboratory conditions of induced hypoxia/asphyxia in primate models, severe asphyxia rarely causes brain damage *in previously normal subjects.* Either fetal death or intact survival are the common responses, with permanent brain damage the exception (18).

A major but flawed means of judging neonatal condition is the Apgar score. Nelson and Ellenberg (16) studied 390 infants (born between 1959 and 1966) from the Collaborative Perinatal Project with very low Apgar scores (0–3) at 10 minutes or later. Of these infants, 270 died before their first anniversary. Of the remaining 120 infants, 99 were followed closely and 87 were found to be free of disabling cerebral palsy (88%). The remaining 12 children had disabling cerebral palsy (12%). When these infants were examined at 7 years of age, 4 had died of cerebral palsy between the ages of 1 and 7. Of interest, 55% of the children who later developed cerebral palsy had 1-minute Apgar scores of 7–10. Cerebral palsy is 162 times more likely to occur in neonates whose Apgar score is 0–3 at 20 minutes than in infants with a 20-minute score of 4 or greater. However, at least 60% of the surviving neonates with 20-minute Apgar scores of 1–3 do not develop cerebral palsy (19). Thus, even severe and prolonged depression in otherwise normal neonates does not invariably result in long-term disability.

Thompson and colleagues (20) followed 31 children who had 1-minute Apgar scores of 0 or less than 4, at 5 minutes. When examined between 5 and 10 years of age, 29/31 (93%) were found to have no neurologic handicap. Indeed in this series, two children thought to be stillborn at birth were eventually noted to have neurologically normal behavior in the nursery. As may not be surprising from our discussion so far, Sykes and coworkers (21) noted a poor correlation between

Apgar scores and neonatal acidosis. Only 21% of babies with low 1-minute Apgar scores and 19% of babies with low 5-minute Apgar scores had evidence of severe acidosis at birth. Similarly 73% of babies with severe acidosis had a 1-minute Apgar of 7 or greater. 85% had a similar 5-minute score.

There is additional clinical data from humans to support a similar conclusion. In Grausz's series, 42/146 neonatal deaths (28.5%) were attributed to asphyxia (17). However, the incidence of documented asphyxia in obstetrical practice is low. Even in pregnancies longer than 259 days, neonatal asphyxia is observed in less than 1% of cases. Of greater concern to clinicians is asphyxia sufficient to damage but not to kill the fetus/neonate.

We may fairly conclude that even in the most severely depressed neonates, accurately predicting long-term abnormal development is uncertain using current techniques (19, 22–24). Our difficulty is that the early overall neonatal status (which is only partially measured by the Apgar score) *does correlate* with ultimate outcome but our techniques are inaccurate in the prediction of long-term outcome. There is also evidence that the neurologic performance of infants can improve over time despite early evidence suggesting cerebral palsy (19, 25). Thus, brain healing or plasticity must be considered as a confounding variable in the evaluation of an apparently damaged neonate at birth. In sum, firm predictions of eventual permanent damage in depressed or apparently injured neonates are not possible with great accuracy, except in extreme cases.

Despite these limitations, the neonatal Apgar score remains important for the same reasons as when it was initiated by Virginia Apgar in the 1950s. The original intention of the score was to direct the attention of the clinician to the need for immediate neonatal resuscitation. Clinicially, we recognize that the Apgar score most accurately reflects acute events during labor, fetal distress occurring immediately prior to birth, or immediate neonatal events (e.g., suctioning/intubation for meconium). *As the Apgar score documents only one moment in time and because its scoring is in part subjective, the relationship between an abnormal Apgar score and ultimate neonatal fetal brain development is limited.* The implications of Apgar scoring should not be overly extended.

There is evidence that intrapartum asphyxia can be the *result* *rather than the cause* of neurologic abnormality (12). If intrapartum asphyxia were the major cause of subsequent brain injury, then evidence for such asphyxia, including abnormal electronic fetal monitoring patterns, low Apgar scores, and the results of fetal blood sampling suggestive of fetal acidosis, should all be strong and reliable predictors of brain injury, yet they are not. Also, we would expect that the birth histories of most children with cerebral palsy should reveal evidence of intrapartum or newborn asphyxia, yet many do not (13, 15). Therefore, the mere presence of documented hypoxia/asphyxia during the intrapartum period does not certify a cause and effect relationship between that hypoxia/asphyxia and subsequent brain dysfunction. We must not fall into the *post hoc, ergo propter hoc* fallacy in our thinking about cerebral palsy and other types of neonatal brain dysfunction.

If we disregard this argument so far and conclude that evidence of fetal acidosis or asphyxia as diagnosed by a scalp sampling, electronic fetal monitoring, etc. reliably predicts fetal asphyxia/acidosis and that such asphyxia leads to fetal brain injury, a possibility exists for reducing the risk of such injury by obstetric intervention when abnormal patterns are recognized. However, it is uncertain whether intrapartum obstetric intervention to avoid asphyxia actually reduces the risk of neonatal brain injury. Based on available data, it is reasonable to argue that the injury was already present in many cases when the fetal asphyxia was recognized (i.e., the already sick fetuses are the ones likely to get into trouble with abnormal decelerations, bradycardia, etc.). Similarly, the effects of asphyxia may or may not be reversible.

These are important considerations for clinical practice (9). Obstetric procedures, including instrumental delivery, can be beneficial or harmful to mother and child. Unfortunately, patients (and clinicians) have developed unrealistic expectations of what prenatal and antepartum interventions can accomplish or prevent. As obstetricians we are open to the charge that we have oversold both ourselves and the general public on the accuracy and predictability of our diagnostic techniques and the invariable, beneficial effects of our interventions. A good example here is cesarean delivery for breech presentation fetuses regardless of gestational age or condition. It is difficult and probably not possible to prove that this increased rate of operative delivery for the majority of breech presentation fetuses has resulted in any demonstrable improvement in the long-term outcome of these infants. A most careful, critical analysis of obstetric interventions is in order for us to retain both our clinical credibility and control our medicolegal risks in modern practice.

Importance of Antepartum Events: Overview

It is the belief of many obstetricians/gynecologists (and the general public) that most brain damage results from events during labor and delivery. However, this simply is not true (12, 13, 15). Genetic, social, and many other factors are more appropriate etiologies for severe brain damage (cerebral palsy). It is clear that the role of perinatal events in cerebral palsy is often overestimated (12, 13, 26). Although it is true that many cases of cerebral palsy are related to perinatal events, as we have seen, at least 50% of neonates who are later diagnosed as having cerebral palsy are not depressed at the time of birth, at least as reflected in Apgar scores.

Serious physical trauma in obstetric practice is uncommon in modern management. Heroic procedures are in general avoided and intrapartum management is increasingly sophisticated (23). However, or we have seen, intrapartum asphyxia and, to a much lesser extent, intrapartum trauma contribute to neonatal morbidity. Other factors, including disordered fetal growth, prematurity, intrauterine infection, and chromosomal and other nongenetic congenital abnormalities, outweigh intrapartum asphyxia as contributors to brain damage and poor long-term neonatal development (13, 15). For example, severe mental retardation relates to prenatal genetic and/or chromsomal problems in some 70% of cases (13). These facts have led to increasing attention to antepartum asphyxia characterized by biochemical events leading to tissue ischemia and/or hemorrhage as a cause for severe brain damage.

The importance of antenatal factors in contributing to neonatal morbidity needs special emphasis. Acute perinatal risk factors, including trauma, asphyxia, hyperbilirubinemia, or hypoglycemia, occur in only about 8% of severely mentally retarded children (23). In an analysis of etiologic factors in cerebral palsy and severe mental retardation, Durkin et al. (27) found an increased incidence of prematurity, postmaturity, large for gestational age, maternal diabetes, and mothers older than 35 or younger than 20 years. In 281 cases of mentally retarded patients who had no motor symptoms or cerebral palsy, one-third of the brain damaged children had normal histories. One-third of the patients had problems that were not usually considered to place them at risk for brain damage and only one-third of the mothers had histories that were felt to be responsible or closely related to cerebral palsy.

There is increasing evidence that permanent brain injury is caused by chronic asphyxia or repeated acute episodes superimposed on chronic asphyxia rather than any single, acute asphyxial perinatal episode (9, 16, 23, 28). Thus, diagnosing perinatal asphyxia at a given point during labor may not identify the potentially injured fetus unless the asphyxia occurs in a setting of chronic insufficiency. There is some clinical evidence to support this hypothesis (29). Neonates born to preeclampic women with chronically low estriols are more likely to be abnormal neurologically on follow-up than neonates with either normal estriol levels or acutely dropping levels (30). Recent study of growth-retarded fetuses by transcutaneous direct umbilical vessel blood sampling has documented advanced asphyxia. In some instances the blood gas abnormalities have developed prior to labor (31).

In sum, there is evidence that limited risk of brain damage exists in previously normal but acutely asphyxiated newborns when compared to nonasphyxiated children *unless* the asphyxiated neonate has suffered some form of chronic prenatal deprivation (intrauterine growth retardation, uteroplacental insufficiency of postdatism pregnancy, chronic maternal hypertensive disease, etc.).

Importance of Intrapartum Events: Immediate Trauma

The clinical use of forceps or the vacuum extractor carries an increased risk of both maternal and neonatal trauma (see Chapter 5). To determine the true incidence of various injuries, however, is a difficult task due to vast differences in study design and reporting. Further, complications of instrumental delivery are not entirely procedure-dependent, but also involve elements of operator skill and training. These factors complicate any assessment of risk. Evaluation of the status of the neonate is also difficult. Infants requiring assisted delivery are more likely to prove abnormal than infants from uncomplicated labors, independent of the process of delivery. Therefore, relating adverse neonatal status completely to the use of forceps or the vacuum extractor is both inaccurate and misleading. Some studies, however, have attempted to draw such impossible conclusions.

Chiswick and James (32) compared 86 babies delivered by Kielland forceps (or by emergency cesarean section after an attempted Kielland forceps delivery) to 86 babies born spontaneously. Outcome measures of delayed onset response, birth trauma, abnormal neurological behavior, and jaundice were used. These authors found all these events to be significantly more frequent among the forceps delivery group in comparison to their controls. However, drawing such conclusions is not valid, especially in light of the finding that 56% of the forceps deliveries were performed for a prolonged second stage of labor, 19% for prolonged second stage and fetal asphyxia, and 17% for fetal asphyxia alone. It is illuminating to compare the study of Chiswick and James to one where a more appropriate comparison group has been chosen. For example, Dierker and coworkers (8) compared midforceps deliveries to all deliveries and then *specifically to infants delivered by cesarean section for similar clinical indications.* They concluded that the judicious use of midforceps is not associated with increased short-term risk. Although 1-minute Apgar scores were significantly lower and the incidence of cephalhematomas were significantly higher in those infants delivered by midforceps as compared to the entire study population, there were no significant differences in short-term neonatal morbidity in the midforceps cases *when matched to infants delivered by cesarean section.* Those authors state that the matched groups appear to represent fetuses at risk for some abnormal short-term outcome, unrelated to the delivery method. Thus, not only did the study of Chiswick and James use an inappropriate control group (subjects delivered by normal spontaneous vaginal delivery), but it did not address other important characteristics of labor or delivery that may have affected neonatal performance. Studies done by Benaron and coworkers (33) and Wetterdal (34) have the same shortcomings. These arguments do not obscure the fact that in a small percentage of cases instrumental delivery clearly produces fetal (and maternal) trauma. Fortunately, the vast majority of injuries are of minor clinical consequence, although some can be serious and rarely even fatal (see Chapter 5).

Importance of Intrapartum Events: Long-term Complications

Critical evaluation of the literature and comparing results becomes a complex and frustrating task when long-term complications of instrumental delivery are considered. Study design and data collection are greatly disparate. Many "studies" in the literature are in effect clinical testimonials, absent of properly chosen methodology and controls. Unfortunately, much of the available data falls into this category. Amiel-Tison (35) attempted to look at labor and delivery factors that could explain cerebral damage. That author, however, includes but two cases of "difficult forceps." Corston (36) endeavored to determine whether the use of high or midforceps impaired later physical or mental development. Although the study did not conclude that forceps-delivered subjects had impaired IQs, it is not possible to draw any meaningful conclusions from the data.

A potentially good study can also become totally useless simply because the authors neglected to present the total number of controls, making statistical evaluation impossible. Other data can be made difficult to interpret because of the low incidence of some complications. For example, Bowes and Bowes (37) compared the incidence of neonatal morbidity in low versus midforceps procedures and also compared morbidity in midforceps deliveries to patients delivered by the Malmström vacuum extractor or cesarean section in whom the second stage of labor was 2 hours or more. Their data indicate a higher incidence of significant neonatal complications in midforceps deliveries as compared to low forceps, cesarean section, or vacuum extraction deliveries. However, this conclusion cannot be verified because of the small number of total cases.

The single most important factor for a good study evaluating the safety of the forceps operation is the choice of an appropriate control group. However, other design factors also rank high in importance. For example, a proper stratification of the data by various labor and delivery factors is crucial to an appropriate and accurate appraisal. Unfortunately, even among the better studies there are few that are without flaws when closely examined.

Three studies fall slightly short of appropriate design factors, again making it difficult to draw definitive conclusions from their data. Zachau-Christiansen and Villumsen (38) studied 9125 deliveries. Three hundred and thirty-six of these were single births delivered by vacuum extraction and 98 were births delivered by forceps. These were compared to a control group of 915 normal spontaneous vaginal deliveries. All were followed up for 1 year. Attention was directed to signs of fetal distress, including evidence of asphyxia at birth and incidence of neonatal and neurological signs and symptoms. Follow-up studies at 1 year included studies of sitting, crawling, walking, and a series of normal neurological motor behavior. Particular attention was given to noting evidence of neurologic, psychiatric, and motor retardation. These authors observed that the forceps-delivered group were slightly deficient in motor skills at 8 months and at 1 year. However, they also found that the forceps-delivered group included more pregnancies complicated by instances of fetal distress and asphyxia at birth. Thus, it is difficult to sort out which factor or factors was most contributory to the infants' observed abnormalities.

Studies done by Nelson and Broman (39) and Nichols and Chen (40) have the same deficiences and similar conclusions. Nelson and Broman (39) studied motor and mental handicaps in a cohort of individuals born between 1959 and 1966 who were followed until 7 years of age. They examined labor and delivery factors associated with moderate to severe motor and mental handicaps. Bradycardia in the second stage of labor, arrested progress of labor, and the use of midforceps were identified with a higher incidence of long-term problems; however, due to study design they were unable to weigh the relative importance of each. Nichols and Chen (40) found other factors contributing to neonatal damage to be maternal diabetes, fetal brady-cardia during the first stage of labor, vaginal bleeding at admission for delivery, abnormal presentation, low placental weight, and short cord. Without stratifying for each of these factors, it becomes impossible to determine if midforceps operation is the primary or responsible factor in a difficult and complicated case or simply a fellow traveler.

The issue of the role of instrumentation in long-term injury is best addressed by a handful of good studies. For example, Nilsen (41) in Norway performed a follow-up study at 18 years of age of 62 males delivered by forceps versus 38 by vacuum extraction drawn from a total cohort ($N = 31,093$) of military conscripts in 1981 (all 18 years of age). At birth there were no significant differences between the forceps and vacuum extraction groups in terms of gestational age, birth weight, birth length, placental weight, nulliparity, or induction or labor. How-ever, more instances of bradycardia were observed in the forceps group versus the vacuum extraction group. At age 18 no significant differ-ences between the groups were noted in physical morbidity as sur-veyed with a review of systems. In terms of IQ, forceps-delivered males had significantly higher IQs at age 18 than the total conscripts while those men originally delivered by vacuum extraction did not differ from the national average. Of the forceps, 37/62 (59.7%) were outlet operations and there was a significantly higher IQ among this group. Midforceps contributed 29% (18/62), all with rotation, yet they still had significantly higher IQs over the controls; 11.3% (7/62) had been delivered by high forceps, a number too small to calculate mean IQ values.

Broman and coworkers (42) reported an apparent protective effect of prophylactic outlet forceps in conducting a study examining events in labor and delivery as probably causes of neurologic damage. Correlations were sought between neonatal IQ scores and 30 obstetri-cal variables. The study included 1199 white and 2131 black patients. These authors observed that the use of forceps was positively associ-ated with the duration of second stage of labor. There was a negative relationship between outlet and low forceps use, parity and gravity. IQ was analyzed in children at 4 years of age. A positive correlation was noted between IQ scores and the use of forceps. Outlet and midforceps use had a slightly higher IQ than children delivered without the use of forceps. White children who had spontaneous deliveries had IQ scores about 4 points lower than those of children born with forceps from any class. While these authors observed a positive effect of forceps delivery valid conclusions cannot be drawn from these data because, as above, the neonates in the nonoperative delivery group should have been compared to groups of neonates with operative deliveries performed for similar clinical indications.

Reviewing data from the Collaborative Perinatal Project study which included 15,308 black and 14,269 white patients, Niswander and Gordon (10) found that the prophylactic low forceps operation was associated with lower perinatal mortality and better subsequent motor and intellectual function than true for those spontaneously delivered. All of these women were delivered of a single fetus either spontaneously or by low forceps. Excluded from analysis were unattended deliveries, deliveries associated with fetal deaths occurring during labor, pregnancies with fetuses of birth weights less than 1500 g, gravidas with maternal complications of diabetes or acute or chronic hypertensive vascular diseases and certain accidents of pregnancy (abruptio placentae, placenta previa, and prolapse of the umbilical cord). Primigravidas with the second stage greater than 2½ hours or multiparas with the second stage greater than 1½ hours were also excluded. The study was controlled for race, parity, length of second stage of labor, birth weight, and education of the gravida. Outcome measures included the neonatal death rate, the 1 and 5 minute Apgar scores, the 8-month score achieved on the Baley Scales of mental and motor development, 4-year fine motor scores, gross motor scores, and the Stanford-Binet IQ score. Niswander and Gordon concluded that prophylactic low forceps operations resulted in lower perinatal mortality than that associated with spontaneous delivery. Further, prophylactic low forceps operations appeared to exert a favorable effect on the subsequent motor and intellectual function of the children so delivered.

McBride and coworkers (43) compared low, mid, and midforceps with rotation to those delivered by cesarean section or spontaneously. All forceps-delivered infants had a slightly higher IQ at the age of 5. However, stepwise multiple linear regression revealed that family background variables were the most powerful predictors of intellectual ability in the child and that perinatal descriptors and delivery method did not contribute significantly to intellectual ability, at least as measured by IQ testing.

The issue of long-term outcome following instrumental delivery is most prominently argued by Dierker et al. (7, 8) and Friedman et al (5, 6). Freidman and coworkers first addressed the issue in the late 1970s (5). They studied 1194 patients for whom well-documented labor progression patterns were available. A total of 656 of the neonates from these deliveries were evaluated intensively at 3 and 4 years of age with a battery of speech and hearing tests. IQ scores were obtained. The population included 263 infants delivered spontaneously, 168 by low forceps, 181 by midforceps, 16 by cesarean section, 24 by assisted breech delivery, and 4 delivered by version and breech extraction. The authors controlled for race and parity, and stratified the data for labor patterns according to the types of delivery. Mean IQ scores appeared to be correlated with delivery procedure. The lowest scores occurred among those children delivered vaginally with breech presentation or by midforceps. The best IQ scores occurred among those delivered spontaneously or by low forceps, with children from the spontaneous vaginal deliveries fairing somewhat better than those delivered instrumentally. The authors claimed that both aberrant labor *and* operative vaginal delivery operated independently. That is, labor problems and especially midforceps operations appeared to be associated with significantly lower IQ scores. The midforceps effect reportedly was exerted uniformly without regard for the labor pattern although there was a trend (but not of statistical significance) suggesting a further worsening of fetal condition when the labor curve indicated an arrest disorder. With arrest disorders, there was a uniform lowering of IQ scores in instrumentally delivered infants, regardless of the type of delivery. (Note: only one infant had been delivered spontaneously in this subgroup).

These findings are unique. IQ trends were essentially independent in that both aberrant labor *and* operative deliveries were associated with significantly lower IQ scores. Otherwise stated, it appears as though midforceps exerted a negative effect on IQ scores independent of labor pattern.

A later study by Friedman et al. (6) had similar results. The authors asked the question whether infants delivered by midforceps did as well as infants delivered by other methods when matched case by case. For this study the definition of midforceps was instrumentation for delivery in which the forceps were applied when the fetal head was not on the pelvic floor, i.e., caput was not visible between contractions without spreading the labia or in which the sagittal suture of the fetal head was not in the anteroposterior direction. Thus, rotation regardless of station and any procedure beyond simple outlet forceps was considered a midpelvic procedure. The data in the study was derived from the data bank of the National Cooperative Perinatal Project and included a follow-up of 7 years on the neonates. Neonatal data included IQ measured by the Stanford-Binet intelligence scales. Cases were stratified by race, parity, birth weight, labor pattern, and delivery outcome. Midforceps cases were compared to those delivered spontaneously. While the authors fairly concluded from their data that infants delivered by midforceps had significantly lower mean intelligence quotient as compared to those delivering spontaneously, the matching of patients is in question. It seems more appropriate to match midforceps deliveries with cesarean section deliveries *for the same clinical indications.* This is based on the assumption that cases in each of these categories represent cases at risk, among whom some sort of intervention is indicated. A more accurate appraisal thus becomes possible when additional intrapartum factors such as oxytocin augmentation, fetal heart rate abnormalities, scalp pH, or presence of meconium are examined.

Dierker and coworkers (7) explored the relationship between the "conservative" use of midforceps and neonatal and maternal morbidity. In a subsequent study, Dierker et al. (8) attempted to determine whether the use of forceps resulted in an increase in long-term neurologic morbidity when instrumented pregnancies were compared with a matched group of neonates delivered by cesarean section. For the purposes of this retrospective study, midforceps deliveries were defined as deliveries in which instrumental delivery was performed, while the vertex was engaged but the fetal skull was above the perineum. Excluded from study were infants with major congenital anomalies, multiple gestations, and stillbirths. The cesarean delivery cases were matched to midforceps cases on the basis of the clinical diagnosis of dystocia *and* fetal heart rate recordings suggestive of fetal distress. Cases were also matched for birth weight, gestational age, fetal sex, and race. The neonatal follow-up was for a minimum of 2 years. This two-part study concluded that the conservative use of midforceps is *not* associated with increased neonatal morbidity or adverse, long-term sequelae, as compared to infants delivered by cesarean section for similar indications. The authors found that those delivered by midforceps had significantly more labor abnormalities, including a prolonged latent phase, active protraction, active arrest, protraction of descent, arrest of descent, and a longer second stage of labor. Midforceps deliveries were also associated with more abnormal fetal heart rate patterns. Indications for use of midforceps were fetal distress in 37% of the cases, and dystocia in 38%. What these authors address and what is immediately obvious is that it *seems appropriate to match midforceps deliveries with cesarean deliveries of similar indication with similar evidence of initial fetal condition in judging the appropriateness of a method of delivery.* In midpelvic arrest, when delivery is indicated, the obstetrician has two choices—either cesarean section or instrumental delivery. In this setting, spontaneous vaginal delivery is no longer an option. Thus, in consideration of risks and benefits we should compare the results of assisted vaginal delivery against its only realistic alternative, abdominal delivery. While Friedman and colleagues do address labor abnormalities, their comparison group consisted of infants requiring no assistance at delivery. It is unlikely that the degree of labor difficulty and resultant stress on the neonate would have been as severe in this subgroup.

The etiology of cerebral palsy deserves separate attention. Several authors have attempted to relate it to the use of forceps. In most cases, however, the studies are poor and no definitive conclusions can be drawn. Also confounding the picture is the fact that many of the infants in question are premature, which is known to be the most significant factor influencing the incidence of cerebral palsy. Bishop and coworkers (11) concluded that early and generous episiotomy, followed by gentle outlet forceps, actually protects against the excessive birth trauma. Fuldner (44) examined the birth and neonatal records of 204 children with homogenous central nervous system involvement. He retrospectively found an increased incidence of labor complications, such as persistent malposition, breech presentation, arrest of labor, mid and high forceps application, and premature separation of the placenta. While forceps application may have been contributory, it was not possible to identify the single most important etiologic factor. Mukherjee and coworkers (45) found that 7 of 33 cases felt to have an antenatal origin for their cerebral palsy had been delivered by forceps. They concluded that forceps can be contributory since 21% of the cases were associated with forceps. However, Steer and Bonney (46) found no significant increase in the use of forceps among 317 patients with cerebral palsy. It simply is not possible to draw any definitive conclusions from such reports. Properly designed case control studies are in order for an appropriate appraisal.

Recommendations

What, if any, conclusions can be drawn from these data? First, the judicious use of instrumental delivery is not associated with unacceptable neonatal morbidity. The majority of immediate neonatal injuries are minor and of cosmetic consequence only. Prophylactic outlet forceps operations can fairly be associated with a slightly improved neonatal outcome, although these data are controversial. It can also be argued that in general low and midforceps, when used properly, are associated with favorable outcome, or at least a neutral one if the comparison is made between truly comparable control groups. In terms of the choice of instrument for assisted delivery in various clinical settings, the following outline is suggested.

Outlet Delivery

When assistance in a true outlet delivery (sagittal suture mildine, scalp visible between the labia between contractions, fetal cranium on the pelvic floor) is required, forceps are the instrument of choice. Correctly applied, forceps result in less maternal/fetal trauma for this indication than the principal alternative, the vacuum extractor. While the vacuum extractor might be used in this setting, the classic Malmström instrument risks a cephalhematoma and produces the cosmetically unfavorable chignon. Unfortunately, it is in the outlet application that the least traumatic vacuum extractor, the silastic flexible cup instrument, is most likely to fail.

Trial of Vaginal Delivery

When a true midpelvic extraction is attempted as a trial, the author prefers the vacuum extractor. Difficult rotational midpelvic procedures have no place in modern obstetric management. If station cannot be made with the vacuum extractor, the procedure is terminated and cesarean delivery performed. For trials of instrumental delivery in the lower pelvis, forceps are preferable although the vacuum extractor may also be attempted.

Fetal Distress

In instances of true, acute fetal distress—e.g. cord prolapse, late abruptio placentae—the author favors the use of forceps over the vacuum extractor. Preparations for cesarean delivery are undertaken during an attempt, unless the fetal head is on the perineum. In general, European experience to the contrary, in most clinical settings in the United States forceps can be applied more rapidly than the vacuum extractor due to the ready availability of forceps in all delivery rooms and many years of familiarity with the instruments.

Occiput Posterior Positions

In occiput posterior positions that fail to spontaneously rotate and require assistance, a forceps delivery, face to pubis, is the first preference. Vacuum extraction from the posterior may also be attempted, with the advantage that approximately one-half will rotate anteriorly either spontaneously or with digital assistance (47). If the operator is experienced and delivery as a posterior is not easy, forceps rotation to an anterior position by a modified Scanzoni maneuver is frequently surprisingly simple. Such procedures should not be attempted by the neophyte (48, 49).

Midpelvic Arrests

Vacuum extraction or manual rotation with secondary application of a forceps is equally preferable for most practitioners. Those skilled in midpelvic application of the Kielland or Barton forceps can also apply these instruments with acceptable results (48, 49).

Delivery of the Second Twin

High pelvic delivery of a second, cephalic presentation twin at or near term is a good indication for the use of the vacuum extractor (50). An advantage of the vacuum cup is that it can easily and safely be applied to the cranium of the second twin at higher station than forceps. Below the midpelvis, the instruments are equally useful. At lower station, which instrument is applied depends upon the preference of the operator.

Breech Presentations

This setting is a clear indication for the application of forceps. In near term breech presentations, Piper forceps are the instrument of choice (49). In the setting of vaginal delivery of a preterm breech presentation, which instrument to apply, if any, is less clear (48). The best compromise is likely the application of a small or "baby" forceps, if such are available.

Premature Delivery

The use of any instrument in the delivery of a premature infant is highly controversial. The author favors gentle assisted delivery of the fetal head *on the perineum* using an Elliot-type classic forceps, as there is some evidence that this may reduce cranial trauma. This point is, however, not settled and any such application should be considered elective (48, 49). Here the vacuum extractor is contraindicated.

And here I cease to write, but will not cease
To wish you live in health, and die in peace;
And ye our physic rules that friendly read,
God grant that physic you may never need.
Regimen Sanitatis Salernitanum
ca. 1250 AD (51)

REFERENCES

1. Freud S. Infantile cerebral paralysis. Russin LA (translator). Coral Gables, Florida: University of Florida Press, 1968: 142.
2. Mesmer FA. Dissertatio physico - medica de planetarum influxu vindobonae. Vienna: Ghelen, 1766.
3. Richardson OR, Evans MI, Cibils LA. Midforceps delivery: a critical review. Am J Obstet Gynecol 1983; 145:621–632.
4. Varner MW. Neuropsychiatric sequelae of midforceps deliveries. Clin Perinatol 1983; 10:455–460.
5. Friedman EA, Sachtleben MR, Bresky PA. Dysfunctional labor XII. Long-term effects on infant. Am J Obstet Gynecol 1977; 127:779–783.
6. Friedman EA, Sachtleben-Murray MR, Dahrough D, Neff RK. Long-term effects of labor and delivery on offspring: a matched-pair analysis. Am J Obstet Gynecol 1984; 150:941–945.
7. Dierker LJ, Rosen MG, Thompson K, Debanne S, Linn P. The midforceps: maternal and neonatal outcomes. Am J Obstet Gynecol 1985; 152:176–182.
8. Dierker LJ, Rosen MG, Thompson K, Lynn P. Midforceps deliveries: long-term outcome of infants. Am J Obstet Gynecol 1986; 154:764–768.
9. Niswander KR. Labor and operative obstetrics, asphyxia in the fetus and cerebral palsy. In: Obstetrics and Gynecology. Chicago: Year Book, 1983: 107–125.
10. Niswander KR, Gordon M. Safety of the low-forceps operation. Am J Obstet Gynecol 1973; 117:619–630.
11. Bishop EH, Israel SL, Briscoe CC. Obstetric influences on the premature infants first year of development. Obstet Gynecol 1965; 26:628–635.
12. Illingworth RS. Why blame the obstetrician? A review. Br Med J 1979; I:797–801.
13. Illingworth RS. A paeditrician asks— why is it called birth injury? Br J Obstet Gynaecol 1985; 92:122–130.
14. Holm VA. The causes of cerebral palsy: a contemporary prospective. JAMA 1982; 247:1473–1477.
15. Nelson KB, Ellenberg JH. Antecedents of cerebal palsy. N Engl J Med 1986; 315:81–86.
16. Nelson KB, Ellenberg JH. Apgar scores as predicators of chronic neurologic disability. Pediatrics 1981; 68:36–44.
17. Grausz JP, Heimler R.. Asphyxia and gestational age. Obstet Gynecol 1975; 62:175–179.
18. Niswander, KR. Does substandard obstetric care cause cerebral palsy? Contemp Obstet Gynecol 1987; 30:42–60.
19. Coulter DL. Neurologic uncertainty in newborn intensive care. N Engl J Med 1987; 316:840–844.
20. Thompson AJ, Searle M, Ressell G. Quality of survival after severe birth asphyxia. Arch Dis Child 1977; 52:620–626.
21. Sykes GS, Molloy PM, Johnson P. Do apgar scores indicate asphyxia? Lancet 1982; I:494–496.
22. Brann AW. Factors during neonatal life that influence brain disorders. United States Washington, DC. Department of Health and Human Services, Public Health Service, NIH Publication no. 85-1149, April 1985: 263–358.
23. Rosen MG. Factors during labor and delivery that influence brain disorders. Washington DC: United States Department of Health and Human Services, Public Health Service, NIH Publication no. 85-1149, April 1985: 237–261.
24. Rosen MG, Bilenker RM, Thompson K. Assessment of developmental time periods and risks of brain damage in the fetus and neonate. J Reprod Med 1986; 31:297–303.
25. Nelson KB, Ellenberg JH. Children

who "outgrew" cerebral palsy. Pediatrics 1982; 69:529–536.

26. Paneth N, Stark RI. Cerebral palsy and mental retardation in relation to indicates of perinatal asphyxia. Am J Obstet Gynecol 1983; 147:960–966.

27. Durkin MV, Kaveggia EG, Pendleton E. Analysis of etiologic factors in cerebral palsy with severe mental retardation. Eur J Pediatr 1976; 123:67–81.

28. Niswander K, Elborne D, Henson G, Chalmers I, Redman C, MacFarland A, Tizard P. Adverse outcome of pregnancy and quality of obstetric care. Lancet 1984; 1:827–830.

29. Naeye RL, Peters EC. Antenatal hypoxia and low IQ values. Am J Dis Child 1987; 141:50–54.

30. Yogman MW, Speroff L, Huttenlocker PR, Kase NG. Child development after pregnancies complicated by low urinary estriol excretion and pre-eclampsia. Am J Obstet Gynecol 1972; 114:1069–1077.

31. Nicolaides KH, Soothill PW, Rodeck CH, Campbell S. Ultrasound-guided sampling of umbilical cord and placental blood to assess fetal wellbeing. Lancet 1986; 1:1065–1067.

32. Chiswick ML, James DK. Kielland's forceps: association with neonatal morbidity and mortality. Br Med J 1979; 1:7–9.

33. Benaron HBW, Brown M, Tucker BE, Wentz V, Yacoryznski GK. The remote effects of prolonged labor with forceps deliveries, precipitate labor with spontaneous delivery, and natural labor with spontaneous delivery on the child. Am J Obstet Gynecol 1953; 66:551–556.

34. Wetterdal P. The prognosis for children delivered by forceps. Acta Obstet Gynecol Scand 1927; 6:349–391.

35. Amiel-Tison C. Cerebral damage in full-term new born: aetiological factors, neonatal status and long-term follow-up. Biol Neonate 1969; 14:234–250.

36. Corston JM. The end results in children delivered by mid or high forceps. Am J Obstet Gynecol 1954; 67:263–267.

37. Bowes WA, Bowes C. Current role of the midforceps operation. Clin Obstet Gynecol 1980; 23:549–557.

38. Zachau-Christiansen B, Villumsen A. Follow-up study of children delivered by vacuum-extraction and by forceps. Acta Obstet Gynecol Scand 1964; 43(suppl 7):31–32.

39. Nelson KB, Broman SH. Perinatal risk factors in children with serious motor and mental handicaps. Ann Neurol 1977; 2:371–377.

40. Nichols PL, Chen TC. Minimal brain dysfunction: a prospective study. Hillsdale, England: Lawrence Erlbaum Associates, 1981.

41. Nilsen ST. Boys born by forceps and vacuum extraction examined at 18 years of age. Acta Obstet Gynecol Scand 1984; 63:549–554.

42. Broman SH, Nichols PL, Kennedy WA. Preschool IQ: prenatal and early development correlates. New York: John Wiley & Sons, 1975.

43. McBride WG, Black BP, Brown CJ, Dolby RM, Murray AD, Thomas DB. Method of delivery and developmental outcome at five years of age. Med J Aust 1979; 1:301–304.

44. Fuldner RV. Labor complications and cerebral palsy. Am J Obstet Gynecol 1957; 74:159–166.

45. Mukherjee A, Bole SV, Varma SK. Cerebral palsy in children. A report of 50 cases. Indian J Pediatr 1971; 38:219–222.

46. Steer CM, Bonney W. Obstetric factors in cerebral palsy. Am J Obstet Gynecol 1962; 83:526–531.

47. Thiery M. Obstetric vacuum extraction. Obstet Gynecol Annu 1985; 14:73–111.

48. Laufe LE. Obstetric forceps. New York: Harper & Row, 1968.

49. Dennon EH. Forceps deliveries. 2nd ed. Philadelphia: FA Davis, 1964.

50. O'Grady JP. Clinical management of twins. Contemp Obstet Gynecol 1987; 29:126–145.

51. Guthrie D. A history of medicine. London: Thomas Nelson & Sons, 1945: 110.

INDEX

Page numbers in *italics* denote figures; those followed by "t" denote tables.